Occupational Therapy:
Foundations for Practice
Models, Frames of Reference and Core Skills

Dedicated to Muriel I. Tarrant-Cunningham FCOT and Angela E. Rivett-De Guingaud FCOT ATDip, Founders and former Co-Principals of the London School of Occupational Therapy

For Churchill Livingstone:
Publisher: Mary Law
Project Development Editor: Mairi McCubbin
Editorial Co-ordination: Editorial Resources Unit
  Copy editor: Andrew Gardiner
Design: Design Resources Unit
Production Controller: Nancy Henry
Sales Promotion Executive: Hilary Brown

Occupational Therapy: Foundations for Practice

Models, Frames of Reference and Core Skills

Rosemary Hagedorn DipCOT SROT DipTCDHEd

Course Director in Occupational Therapy, Crawley College
of Technology, Crawley, UK

CHURCHILL LIVINGSTONE
EDINBURGH LONDON MELBOURNE NEW YORK AND TOKYO 1992

CHURCHILL LIVINGSTONE
Medical Division of Longman Group UK Limited

Distributed in the United States of America by Churchill
Livingstone Inc., 650 Avenue of the Americas, New York,
N.Y. 10011, and by associated companies, branches and
representatives throughout the world.

First published 1992

ISBN 0-443-04540-2

British Library Cataloguing in Publication Data
A catalogue record for this book is available from the
British Library.

Library of Congress Cataloging in Publication Data
A catalog record for this book is available from the Library
of Congress.

Produced by Longman Singapore Publishers (Pte) Ltd.
Printed in Singapore

Preface: about myself

You may feel that this is an unduly egocentric way to begin a book, but every author has a past from which he or she cannot escape. It is impossible to write a book of this kind without bringing to it the ideas, beliefs, blinkers, values and prejudices which one has acquired over the years.

Many authors seem to enjoy playing a kind of detective game with the reader, who must try, by the last page, to have uncovered the author's hidden agenda, philosophy and personal idiosyncrasies.

I wish, in this book, to speak directly to you, the reader, in the hope that you will be challenged to think about what you read, to learn actively, and not to take all my ideas at face value, just because they are in print. To this end, it may be useful to begin by knowing a little about my professional background.

I trained at the London School of Occupational Therapy in the days when it was a private establishment ruled by the two memorable people, Miss Muriel Tarrant and Miss Angela Rivett, who were known with awed affection as 'The Aunts'. Because Miss Tarrant has recently died, and because it is to the impeccable models (real, not theoretical) which they provided that I owe most of my values concerning professionalism, I have dedicated this book to them.

I qualified in 1965 and have since had twenty-five years of continuous practice in the south of England. I worked, to begin with, as a therapist in the physical field and later as District Occupational Therapist, developing services for Mental Health and Mental Handicap, and have finally made the sideways jump into education. I am more comfortable with patients aged ninety than nine, I have no direct clinical experience of working in psychiatry and I have never worked in the community.

My preferred model of practice is now Problem Solving, with a strong bias towards cognitive and developmental approaches and a growing flavour of humanism. However, I cannot entirely shake off my behaviourist and biomechanical roots, since those were the main approaches on which my training was based. That has left me with a liking for clear objectives and structured treatment plans which my colleagues in psychiatry often view as overly prescriptive.

I also strongly believe that occupational therapy should be based on occupations and that the primary core skills of the profession are occupational analysis and the therapeutic application of occupations.

In this study guide I have set out to give a concise and objective description of each of the current models and frames of reference, but I am aware that the above biases in ideas and experience are bound to show through and I have tried to make it clear when I am riding one of my own hobby horses, or using my personal set of concepts.

If I may offer you one of the elaborate analogies of which students know I am fond, I have tried to write a kind of 'tourist guide' in which I have climbed a hill and provided you with a potted description of the views in various directions. For a novice tourist, this will probably suffice. If you

v

want to know more, you will have to climb the hill yourself and see the views first hand, not through my perceptions. You may find, if you do, that what you see is not precisely what I have described, and if you have already travelled a particular route several times, your experience is bound to be richer and more varied than my own. That does not make either of us necessarily 'right' or 'wrong', merely different. It is the differences which make for dynamic and adaptive evolution in an organism or a profession.

As a profession we do not spend nearly enough time talking amongst ourselves about what we actually do and what we really think, unpacking the treatment process, comparing terminologies. At a time when we are more than ever under the microscope and obliged to justify our services, this dialogue is an essential tool in defining our methods, objectives and standards.

Finally, I should like to thank the students on the Crawley In-Service Diploma in Occupational Therapy for stimulating me to produce the original Study Guide on which this book is based, and my colleagues Sarah Chapman, Marion Martin and Claudia Rice for ploughing through the drafts and making constructive comments and additions. Those readers who may have seen the earlier booklet will realise that my ideas have inevitably undergone some development during the production of this book and I hope they will not find the slight changes in terminology and organization confusing.

Arundel, 1991   Rosemary Hagedorn

Contents

1

The theoretical basis for occupational therapy

INTRODUCTION TO THE STUDY GUIDE

There are now many frames of reference and models to guide the practice of occupational therapy. Getting to grips with the concepts and terminology can be bewildering. What is the use of a model? What is the difference between a model and a frame of reference? Which one is appropriate in which circumstance? How does theory relate to what the therapist actually does with the patient or client? Do you have a preferred model — or perhaps several?

The purpose of this study guide is to introduce you to a selection of the models and frames of reference which form the foundations for practice, together with their associated approaches and techniques, and to provide sources which will start you on the track of finding more detailed information. This may save some of the time and frustration expended on chasing elusive specialist references in your nearest library.

This book is intended to form a basic text for students and should also be useful to practising therapists who want to extend their theoretical vocabulary and to take a more analytical approach to their work. It is a book about ideas — the 'whys' and 'whats' of occupational therapy — not about the 'hows' of techniques and practice; for the latter, you will need to refer to some of the other sources which I have listed in the Bibliography and Suggested Reading sections.

How to use this study guide

People have individual styles of learning: use this book in any way which you feel to be helpful, but you may like to try some of the following ideas.

Answer the questions as you read

At intervals there are questions which require you to pause in your reading in order to complete a short task. These are designed to help you to clarify your own ideas and perhaps to test them against the ideas in this book. As the answers — or some discussion of possible answers — may be found later in the book, it is best to complete the questions as you come to them, if you wish to use them in the way they are intended.

Read the summary, then do some additional reading

Each model, frame of reference or approach is summarized and a reading list is provided for further study. Some of these lists are quite long to enable you to read in depth about topics of particular interest or relevance. Do not feel obliged to wade through *all* the recommended reading; none the less this study guide can only provide an introduction to a selection of ideas and there is no substitute for reading around the subject. This is particularly so when I am dealing with the work of individual theorists, whose contributions, inevitably, must be paraphrased and perhaps made less accessible in translation. It is advisable, therefore, to do some additional reading if you intend to put a model into practice.

There is a Bibliography at the end of the book which includes all references used in the text; there is also a Suggested Reading list at the end of each chapter. Authors are listed alphabetically, and their publications given in date order. Books and articles listed as suggested reading relate to specific models, frames of reference or techniques, and are given as useful starting points for exploring the literature; they are not comprehensive lists of all available literature, nor do they include some of the references mentioned in the text which are of peripheral interest (the latter can be found in the Bibliography).

Read a section at a time

This study guide contains a great deal of condensed information. Although I hope that it will stimulate your intellectual curiosity and that you will want to read on, it is probably better to break your reading up into manageable chunks, leaving gaps between 'bites', or you are likely to suffer from the mental equivalent of a bad attack of dyspepsia!

Study with a colleague or in a small group

We are dealing with ideas, and half of the interest and challenge is lost if you only have your own experience against which to test the new information. Throughout the book there are discussion points which you can use to trigger your own thinking, making notes if you like. Better still, try to get a few people together to share opinions and compare concepts. You will not always agree — with them, or with me — but that should make your study more interesting.

Think about the applications

Examples of potential applications are given in the description of each approach but these should be taken only as indications of possibilities, and not in any way seen as 'formulae'. If you can relate case studies within your current experience to a particular model or frame of reference, this will help you to understand the application. Try to find your own relevant examples; perhaps start a file of these to illustrate various approaches. Imagine what might happen if a different approach was to be used in a particular case. Talk about your ideas with others. There is some discussion in the text and sometimes questions are posed, but do not expect me to give you one 'right' answer, because there is almost always more than one, and you may well think of alternatives which I did not consider.

There is no single 'right' answer

That there is no single 'right' answer is an important point when we are dealing with frames of reference and models of practice. It is comfortable to have the intellectual and emotional assurance of 'being right'. However, the further one progresses with study, the more one discovers that such certainties are few and that even apparently immutable facts may, on close inspection, be subject to doubt. Knowledge continually evolves. Being confronted with such uncertainties can give rise to feelings of confusion, annoyance and anxiety — particularly if you are to be assessed on your factual knowledge.

The present state of the art in the area of model building and definition of frames of reference within occupational therapy is still at a relatively primitive level of evolution. It is a characteristic of primitive evolutionary processes that diversity is encouraged, successful patterns being continued and less successful ones eliminated. This process is necessary and healthy in developmental terms, but can be highly frustrating educationally.

You will rapidly discover that ideas are fluid; different authors have different versions. This is very challenging to the student, but it also makes it difficult to write a straightforward account of current ideas.

A prominent American educationalist (Perry 1970) has described the developmental process of learning as nine 'Positions', whereby the student makes the difficult cognitive shift from basic dualism (right v. wrong), then moves in stages up the scale of conceptualization and the development of meaning, while gradually recognizing that it is legitimate for authorities to hold different opinions. Finally, the student acknowledges that one must develop one's own commitments and yet be flexible enough to change them as learning continues throughout life.

Interestingly, Perry also describes defensive mechanisms and 'escape routes' at each level, recognizing that students may fight to hold on to a cherished position because movement is too painful, and that the student may actually 'mourn' for the lost position before passing on to the next. Once you have 'stepped up the ladder' you are also quite likely to reject strongly the ideas you previously held. Whether or not you agree with Perry's conceptual model of learning, it may at least be worth remembering that learning produces affective as well as cognitive responses.

Q Before you read any further, make a list of everything which you think might constitute a model, frame of reference or approach — do not let the terminology bother you at this stage. Do these fall into any natural groupings or patterns? What techniques do you associate with each?

Save your list to compare with my proposed classification which you will find later in this section.

OPPOSING VIEWS OF REALITY

Before you tackle the literature on models and frames of reference, it is important to recognize that there are two fundamentally different philosophical perspectives which underpin the various theories concerning the nature of man and his environment. These are mutually incompatible, and generate fierce arguments between their proponents. Many of the misunderstandings which arise when studying models, or when trying to communicate with people who hold an opposing view, spring from a simple failure to take account of this dichotomy.

These perspectives are called the *reductionist* (*atomist* or *mechanistic*) point of view and the *holistic* (or *organismic*) point of view. These have been described as *metamodels* (Reed 1984) since all other models can be viewed as falling into one or other category, and I will use this term as a convenient shorthand.

The terms given in brackets above are often used interchangeably but they are not true synonyms, and the whole exercise of attempting to put models into neat pigeonholes is liable to over-simplfy some very complex philosophical arguments. None the less, it may be helpful to have a basic understanding of the issues and this necessitates concentrating on broader definitions of the metamodels.

The reductionist generally takes a strictly objective and utilitarian view of concrete reality — a reality which can be broken down into observable components. The whole may be understood by studying the parts. The universe operates by rules or laws which will, ultimately, be discovered.

The holistic viewpoint is subjective; reality is mutable, the perceived world is indivisible; abstract and concrete elements interact and form a *gestalt* — a whole which is greater than the sum of its parts. Each element of a gestalt cannot be understood in isolation from the others.

Linked with these opposing concepts is the ancient debate concerning free will and determinism. Is an individual able to make conscious and rational choices — a view held by most holistic philosophies — or are choices ultimately decided by factors such as environmental conditioning and the effects of past experience?

Another contentious area in philosophy is the argument between those who believe that human beings have both mind (and/or spirit) and body, and that these are separate entities (a theory known as dualism), and those who believe that mind is inseparable from, or a product of, body, (a theory known as monism). Generally one can regard dualists as likely to take an holistic standpoint and monists as taking a reductionist one — but some holistic philosophers believe strongly in the inseparability and close linkage between body and mind, and some mechanists simply disregard mind completely and only deal with body (. . . and after that it really gets complicated!). If you wish to find out more about these ideas you will need to read books on metaphysics.

The main concepts of the two metamodels can be summarized (Table 1), but tempting though it is to make a neat list of opposites, it must be recognized that this involves simplification of highly complex debates and such generalization is inevitably not entirely accurate. A much more detailed discussion and comparison has been produced by Reed (1984).

Some authors are damning about the view which they do not happen to share — I consider that it is preferable to regard the two views non-judgementally as *different*, but equally valid in the appropriate context, rather than as good or bad, right or wrong. But how, you may wonder, can one accept two such contradictory views of reality? You may find the following analogy helpful: imagine that if you climb a mountain and look north, you can see a wide desert plain; turning and looking south, you see fertile valleys running to the sea. Both are parts of the same country, but you cannot look at both at the same time, nor would you journey into each in search of the same natural resources. If you descend the mountain, however, and stand in the centre of one area, for you in this position, the other area ceases to exist. The two differing landscapes are analogous to the two differing views of reality.

> **Q** Think about the differences in Table 1. To which side of the 'great divide' do you belong? How, in practical terms, does an awareness of the incompatibility of these metamodels help the therapist?

Table 1 Comparison of holistic/organismic and reductionist/mechanistic metamodels

Holistic/organismic	Reductionist/mechanistic
Views person as a whole 'greater than the sum of its parts'	Views individual as divisible into components which may be studied separately
Tends to think of systems as interactive and adaptive	Tends to think of systems as closed and fixed
Control is based within the individual, who has free will and can make conscious, rational decisions	Deterministic: control is external to the individual, or has an involuntary basis
Present/future oriented	Past/present oriented
Thoughts, feelings and perceptions are important and affect behaviour	Behaviour is important: thoughts and emotions are by-products of physiology and/or behaviour
Behaviour exceeds the utilitarian	Behaviour is utilitarian
Spirituality can be acknowledged	Spirituality is not usually acknowledged
Subjective methods of research are valid	Objective methods of research are valid

(adapted from Reed 1984)

KEY SCHOOLS OF THOUGHT

Occupational therapists treat people, and the knowledge base of occupational therapy is derived mainly from the biological, medical and social sciences. Occupational therapy (OT) philosophy and practice have evolved from the application of such knowledge. It is therefore useful briefly to review the six key schools of thought, each of which produces a different theory of human behaviour. You will probably recognize these theories as the foundations of some widely used models or frames of reference in OT. (A full discussion of the basic theory in each case will be found in psychology textbooks.)

The key schools of thought can be summarized as follows.

Explanations of behaviour

Physiological: We are what our genes and electrochemical functions make us capable of being.

Psychoanalytical: We are what the unconscious memories of our pasts have made us.

Behavioural: We are what our environment demands of us.

Cognitive: We are what our thoughts and perceptions make us.

Developmental: We are what time and change has enabled us to become.

Humanist: We are what we choose to become.

Physiological and behavioural theories are based on the reductionist point of view. Research follows the principles of *scientific realism* or *logical empiricism*, in which reality is viewed as stable and measurable. It emphasizes the necessity for objective studies under closely controlled experimental conditions, producing replicable results, in order to establish scientific principles or facts about the human body or human behaviour. Such research is quantitative and is expected to produce statistics and carefully proved experimental data. Typical methods are surveys, questionnaires, experiments with control groups and 'blind' and 'double-blind' trials.

Psychoanalytical theories are also reductionist in that they stem from classical Freudian determinism — behaviour is influenced by unconscious drives, memories, past experiences and emotions, which can be analysed. However, the more recent humanist psychoanalytical theories, better classified as *psychotherapy*, emphasize choice and free will, and are holistic.

Cognitive, developmental and humanist theories are holistic. They may also be described as *phenomenological*. This is an umbrella term applied to several different schools of philosophy or psychology. A phenomenological approach takes account of the subjective nature of experience and recognizes the unique and changing nature of this experience for each individual. Research is more usually qualitative than quantitative, and may use *ethnographic* techniques (derived from social science and anthropology), *naturalistic research* or *illuminative studies*. Use will be made of personal experience, descriptions, interviews, recordings, field studies and case studies — all of which are typically hard to replicate and evaluate in strictly scientific terms. (There is an increasing acceptance of the validity of the latter methods in the context of occupational therapy.)

Why are metamodels significant?

You will probably have realized by now that combining techniques which are compatible is likely to be more effective than trying to combine those from opposing perspectives.

For example, behaviourism is reductionist and deterministic. Humanism is holistic and self-actualizing. Using a rigid behavioural modification programme at the same time as a programme emphasizing choice and self-selection would be unlikely to work well as simultaneous treatments for an individual. (Conflicts of this kind are not unknown when different members of a treatment team work from the basis of incompatible models and without adequate discussion.)

It is therefore important to be aware of the underlying philosophy of a model, frame of reference or approach and to ensure that the techniques used are compatible with it and with each other. This is not to say that a skilful and experienced practitioner may not 'break the rules' and succeed in combining apparently incompatible techniques, but this should only be done deliberately and with caution.

Coping with the terminology

One of the chief difficulties for the student confronted by the literature on occupational therapy theory, and who is struggling to obtain a clear conception of the meanings of various terms and their inter-relationships, is the realization that these meanings change from one book to the next.

There is no room in this study guide for a detailed discussion of the complexities of the structure, language and formation of models and frames of reference and the problems of creating a professional taxonomy. Further information on this can be found in the reading references at the end of this chapter.

It is unfortunate that there are not, as yet, standard definitions of descriptive terms and concepts. British and American authors use terms in differing ways, and individual authors also differ from each other. Words are frequently used loosely, or interchangeably. (Perhaps in due course the World Federation of Occupational Therapists will provide us with an agreed list of standard terminology?)

The terms *paradigm, model, frame of reference* and *approach* are those which cause the most difficulty. Differing definitions abound and it is clear that within the profession, we have not reached a consensus about how these should be used.

There *is* consensus that the various terms operate at differing conceptual or organizational levels, and have differing functions. The main area of disagreement seems to be over the way in which terms relate to each other. Some authors attribute a conceptual 'weighting' to the various terms, some use several in an heirarchical manner, others use only two, and yet others attribute far more complex relationships.

I have attempted to reflect what I believe to be the current majority view of usage, and I have given a number of definitions in the Glossary so that you can reach your own decision. The organizational scheme which I have chosen to use for

this book is described later in this chapter. A detailed presentation of all the available structures is also beyond the scope of this study guide. For this, you will need to read the original sources listed at the end of this chapter. A few other terms which cause confusion are defined and explained below. For other definitions, refer to the Glossary (p. 87).

Paradigm

With the exception of Mosey (1986) and authors who follow her terminology (i.e. those who use 'model' in a similar sense to the way in which 'paradigm' is used by others), there appears to be quite good agreement about what the *function* of a paradigm should be — that is, to provide a single statement of the fundamental principles and philosophy upon which a profession is based.

There is less agreement about the definition of the word — perhaps because there are, in fact, varied usages in the scientific literature. There is also disagreement over whether or not occupational therapy possesses a defined paradigm. The majority view is that it is probably still developing one, but Creek (1990) has proposed an occupational therapy paradigm. She defines the term as 'an agreed body of theory explaining and rationalizing professional unity and practice, that incorporates all the profession's concerns, concepts and expertise and guides values and commitments'. Another version (Kielhofner 1988) states that it is 'a consensus of the most fundamental beliefs or assumptions of a field'.

Whether or not the profession has yet achieved a paradigm, there are several definitions of occupational therapy which share the common theme of the importance of occupations in promoting and sustaining healthy and meaningful human life, and their potential use as therapy. It may be that an occupational therapy paradigm, when eventually decided, will relate to these fundamental elements of the profession.

Frame of reference and model

The attempts to distinguish between *frame of reference* and *model* constitute a semantic minefield, as may be seen by comparing the quotations below.

In summary, model building is composed of five phases which form a sequence of interlocking systems . . . the frame of reference, assumptions and concepts are crucial to exploring, organizing and developing the model. . . . [A frame of reference is] a mechanism which can be used to explain the relationship of theory to action . . . [it] is not the total model, but does form part of the model building process (Reed 1984).

Although professions have only one model, they usually have a variety of frames of reference . . . [which] derive from a profession's model, and provide guidance on day to day interaction with clients. A frame of reference is far more limited than a model (Mosey 1986).

A frame of reference refers to principles behind practice with a specific patient or client population. It includes a statement of the population to be served, guidelines for determining adequate function or dysfunction and principles for remediation (Bruce & Borg 1987).

Within each frame of reference, one or more models has developed to give more specific direction to practice in the various areas in which occupational therapists work (Creek 1990).

In these circumstances, confusion in the mind of the student is legitimate and one can only sympathize with authors who invent their own terminology: 'We use the terms "theoretical framework" and "theory" in this paper to connote "theory", "model" and "theoretical approach" because the latter terms have no accepted definitions in the profession' (Javatz & Katz 1989).

If you find it impossible to cope with all the arguments over words at this stage, it may be comforting to know that you are not alone in this feeling. Use the terminology with which you are most comfortable: you will probably find at least one authority to support you! However, you would be wise to ascertain which definition an author is employing before begining to study a text.

An attempt to find a unifying definition for each term at this stage is probably either brave or foolhardy, but since I cannot write this study guide on the basis of continual 'ifs and buts', I have decided on the following interpretations.

> **Frame of reference** a framework which draws together the unifying theories and hypotheses of an area of study or practice and sets boundaries to, and foundations for, the construction of models and approaches.
>
> **Model** a statement of an organized and synthesized body of knowledge which demonstrates relationships between elements within the model and between theory and practice, and coordinates the application of relevant approaches and techniques.

Approach

This word tends to be applied rather more loosely and is less well defined than the other terms. It is generally used to describe a set of ideas and actions which provide the therapist with a particular focus which will lead to the selection of specific assessments, media, treatment techniques, or a style of relationship with the patient/client. Approaches are therefore closely related to techniques and methods and differ from frames of reference in that they are narrower, and from models in that they lack the latters' depth of conceptualization and integrative or organizing function. To put it another way, frames of reference and models propose 'what and why', whereas approaches describe 'what and how' (and, possibly, 'to whom'). Since the term *approach* has been extensively used in this study guide, it may be helpful to define it more precisely at this point.

One needs some criteria by which to decide whether or not one is justifed in calling a style of practice an approach. My own test is that an approach should:

- have boundaries to the content. It should possess a definable and coherent set of concepts which are distinctly different from other sets.
- be directive and exclusive. It should oblige one to think and act in a circumscribed manner when working within it, excluding ideas and actions which are incompatible or irrelevant.
- enable a clear definition of the patient's or

client's problem to be made. It should provide an explanation for the origin of the client's dysfunction or need, and provide consequent guidance on appropriate action.
- have defined methods of practical application. It should provide one with a related set of assessment and treatment techniques which are used in a specific way within it.
- include a unique definition of outcome. It should enable the practitioner to judge success or failure within the context of the approach.

I have used this term principally to describe the means whereby theory is translated into practice. For example, a behaviourist frame of reference produces a package of ideas and potential actions which can be called a behaviourist approach. This package very clearly excludes a large number of other possible ideas and actions which would be incompatible or irrelevant. It also includes a range

---

Are you still muddled about the use and meaning of these terms?

If you are, do not worry — you can understand the rest of this study guide without needing to be too precise about the distinctions between terms, and your understanding of them will probably become clearer as you read on. If you disagree with me and have become used to different definitions, stick with them for the moment and review whether you wish to change your views later.

It may help you to relate the terms to a more familiar concept: that of designing a house.

You start with a general concept of a house: it must have a floor, roof, walls and various rooms. You may choose to include the ideas of an apartment or bungalow in your definition, but you will probably decide that a tent or a caravan are not 'houses' in the usual sense of the word.

This is your **paradigm**. It tells you what OT is about and helps you to decide what is, or is not, OT.

A house may contain various rooms — kitchen; bathroom; living room; cellar; attic; nursery; etc. Each contains different furniture and appliances and has a different purpose. Some of the above rooms will be useful to you, others may not.

The rooms are your **frames of reference**. You can choose to use the ones which are appropriate.

Now you can design a particular **kind** of house: you will select a size and shape suited to your special purposes, and will choose to include certain rooms and to leave others out.

This is your **model**. It brings certain ideas together and excludes others.

Finally, you can move into your house and start to live there. At certain times you may use one room and its contents; at others you may move around using different rooms or parts of a room or the appliances within it. However, you can only use what is in the house.

This is your **approach**. You can choose which techniques or media to use, but you can only use the ones which are available within the model or frame of reference you are working with.

of behavioural assessments and behavioural treatment techniques, together with theoretical explanations of behaviour which can be used in the treatment of a patient. Sometimes one frame of reference can generate more than one approach: for example, the physiological frame of reference gives rise to the biomechanical approach and also the neurodevelopmental approach.

Other terms

The following definitions are taken from the Concise Oxford Dictionary (1982).

Philosophy

Seeking after wisdom or knowledge, especially that which deals with ultimate reality or with the most general causes and principles of things and ideas and human perception and knowledge of them

When applied to a profession, philosophy may mean the general beliefs, ideas and knowledge which underpin its practice.

Theory

Supposition or system of ideas explaining something

— is only the first of a number of definitions. The theory sets out the explanation; it includes or assumes facts and phenomena, which may or may not be scientifically or objectively proved — the theory does not deal with such proof. This simple definition is misleading because it ignores a huge philosophical argument about the nature, purpose and validity of theory in general, systems for the construction of theories, and whether a theory can *ever* be proved, or whether it can only be refuted. (For a full discussion of this, ask your librarian for books which summarize the ideas of Popper or Kuhn.) Models combine and show relationships between theories or elements within theories.

Hypothesis

A proposition made as a basis for reasoning without assumption of its truth; a supposition made as a starting point for further investigation of known facts

An hypothesis is usually formulated with a view to testing it out by means of formal research; it may be proved or disproved, or may lead to the formulation of a new hypothesis.

AN ORGANIZATIONAL MODEL

Relationships between elements of professional practice

As already indicated, at the time of writing there is no standard method of classification for frames of reference, models or approaches, nor are the names used to identify each standardized. To avoid tedious repetition I will now refer to these terms in group form as *structures*.

The classification system which I use is my personal system of conceptualization and therefore requires some explanation and justification. There is an important distinction between the organizational model which I present (which you may choose to accept or reject) and the description of each structure, which attempts to present an objective summary of currently accepted thinking. (If you find the classification system and nomenclature inhibiting at first sight, it is probably better to put this aspect to one side and to concentrate on the content rather than the terminology, at least to begin with.)

I consider that professional practice is composed of four related elements. Three of these have al-

---

Frames of reference — provide a statement of facts, theories and hypotheses in a particular field of study.

Models — form a synthesis and integration of elements of theory and practice, derived from various fields of study.

Approaches — form a synthesis of related techniques and methods.

Core skills — basic components of professional practice — managerial, interactive and therapeutic — which remain relatively constant, although adapted by the use of frames of reference, models and approaches.

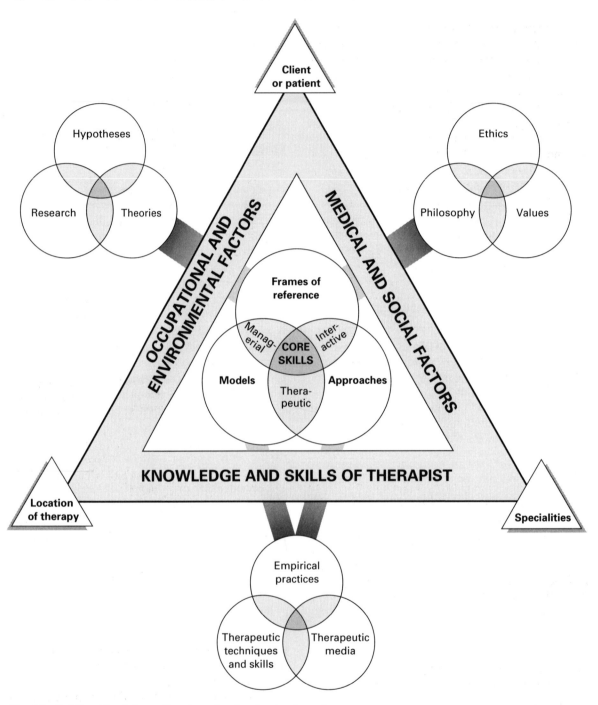

Fig. 1.1 Relationships between the elements of professional practice.

ready been described: frames of reference, models and approaches. The fourth element is the range of core skills of the practitioner, which I describe in Chapter 5 of this book. Each of these elements has a different function (see box on p. 9).

Whilst these terms clearly operate at differing levels of conceptualization and practice, the argument over which came first seems to me as redundant as the cliché 'chicken and egg' debate; all four elements need to be considered holistically, none has meaning without the others.

Figure 1.1 illustrates these relationships.

The theories, hypotheses and research base of the profession combine with the profession's philosophy, values and ethics to produce the basic core skills of the profession, together with frames of reference, models and approaches which direct therapeutic application.

The practice of occupational therapy — empirical experience, developing skills and techniques and the use of therapeutic media is founded on professional core skills and feeds back into models, approaches and frames of reference and their related clinical techniques.

The development, selection and use of core skills, models, frames of reference and approaches is related to the client's occupations and roles, his or her environment, social situation and relevant medical factors; the context, location and environment of therapy is a further factor, together with the knowledge base, style, skills and experience of the individual therapist.

Weighting of any element within the scheme will vary depending on circumstances, although the needs of the client, the core skills of occupational therapy and the overall philosophy of the profession can be expected to exert dominating influences.

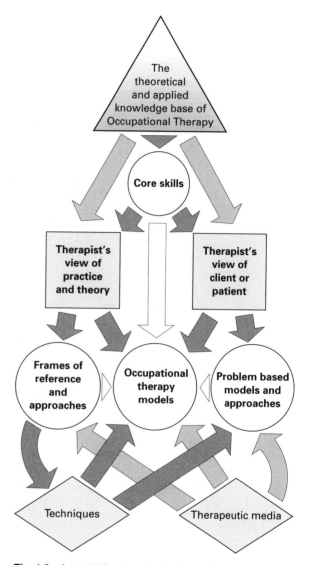

Fig. 1.2 A model for the classification of structures for practice.

Classification of frames of reference, models and approaches

The classification system used in this book is divided into three chapters, one dealing with frames of reference and their associated approaches and techniques, and two with integrative models which serve to coordinate the application of these techniques. A final chapter deals with the core skills of occupational therapy.

This structure is based on the following logic of application. The therapist uses a model or frame of reference to enable her to apply her core skills to the best advantage in treating a patient. When a therapist chooses a model or frame of reference, she does so on the basis of her understanding of the theoretical and applied knowledge base of the profession. This knowledge base produces two distinct perspectives for the therapist:

- A personal view of the core skills, philosophy and practice of the profession;
- A view of the client, identifying the problem and the required intervention.

The first perspective results in the use of frames of reference which are derived from basic theories of human personality and behaviour. From these frames of reference stem many of the approaches and techniques which form the foundation of OT practice.

The second perspective — the view of the client/patient — results in the construction of models related to the perceived nature of the problem, or designed to discover what the nature of the problem may be. These models integrate theories and techniques derived from several frames of reference.

The third group, occupational therapy models, are derived from a synthesis of the two perspectives, and aim to provide an integrative structure for practice which is unique to the profession.

Figure 1.2 shows the structure and its relationship to the two perspectives.

Q Take some time to look at Fig. 1.2 carefully before reading any further. Find your own list of models, frames of reference and approaches which you made earlier. Did you create an organizational model? If so, how does it compare with mine?

Frames of reference

The theoretical bases of these frames of reference are used by a variety of professions, but are applied in a specific way in the context of occupational therapy. It is probable that few therapists work exclusively or strictly within any of these frames (unless in the context of a work environment where a particular frame strongly directs policy), but they have been highly influential in developing distinct approaches and associated

techniques which are frequently used in the context of problem based models and occupational therapy models.

Frame of reference	Approach
• PHYSIOLOGICAL	Neurodevelopmental; Biomechanical
• BEHAVIOURAL	Behavioural
• PSYCHODYNAMIC	Analytical; Interactive
• COGNITIVE	Cognitive
• HUMANIST	Client centred

Problem based models

These models, too, cannot be claimed as being unique to occupational therapy but they are used in a special way within the OT context. They are probably the most commonly used models and are the means by which techniques derived from various therapeutic approaches are integrated.

Rehabilitation

Education

Development

Problem solving

Occupational therapy models

These are all integrative models which seek to form a synthesis of theories to provide an explanation of human behaviour in terms of occupational performance, and as a guide to treatment which is unique to occupational therapy. I have selected three American models which, although not widely used in Britain, have been seminal in raising awareness of the value and scope of integrative models.

Human occupation (Kielhofner)

Adaptive skills (Mosey)

Adaptation through occupation (Reed)

Other structures exist

It is not the purpose of this book to give an account of every possible frame of reference, model or approach. Apart from the fact that this has quite recently been done (Reed 1984), this study guide seeks to represent the current state of practice in Britain, where a more limited range of models and frames of reference is in use. Inevitably, this list can be criticized for its omissions.

You may have decided already that there is one glaring omission — I have not mentioned activities

---

Are you already using a model or frame of reference?

If you are a practising therapist or have had some experience as a student on clinical placements, you have probably already developed, or are in the process of developing, a personal style and a preference for one or more structures. You may already be quite conscious of this, but if not, try answering this short 'quiz'.

			Score (ring code letter)
1	How do you describe your main role?	*Therapist*	a
		Facilitator	b
		Trainer/educator	c
		Resource manager	q
2	How do you refer to the people with whom you deal?	*Patients*	a
		Clients	b
		Trainees/students	c
		Consumers	q
3	Who takes the main decisions about what happens to your patient/client?	*Yourself*	a
		The patient/client	b
		Both of you together	b
		Other person/people (doctor; team)	m
4	What do you see as the main aims of your intervention?	*To regain lost function*	a
		To change behaviour	c
		To inform/educate	e
		To develop potential and abilities	d
		To aid self-actualization	b
		To minimize disability	a
		To train skills	c/e
		To solve problems	f
		To develop insight	g
5	What techniques are you most comfortable with/do you use frequently?	*Creative therapies*	g
		Behaviour modification	c
		Orthotics	a/r
		ADL	a
		Social skills training	c
		Group therapy	g
		Home adaptations	a
		Positioning and reflex inhibition	d
		Specific therapeutic apparatus	a/r

Now count and make a note of the letters you have ringed. (Answers to letter codes are on p. 15.)

or occupations as a basic model or frame of reference. There is a simple reason for this: I consider that models and frames of reference are professional options which one may select or discard as one wishes. The central concern with the analysis and application of occupations and activities and their significance in human life is not such an option: it is the pivot of the profession, results in the use of essential core skills and must be considered as part of occupational therapy's paradigm.

When it comes to nomenclature, we have again, unfortunately, to cope with the problem of lack of standardization. The names of frames of reference, models and approaches used are mainly those which occur frequently in the current literature (Bruce & Borg 1987; Hopkins & Smith 1988; Javetz & Katz 1989; Reed 1984), although I have added a few of my own, either as convenient shorthand, or to cover areas which I believe have been previously omitted from the literature.

SELECTING A STRUCTURE

By now it should be clear there are many available models and frames of reference. How does one avoid becoming totally bewildered and how does one choose the right one for any given situation? In practice it may be less of a difficulty than it appears at first.

- The nature of the patient's problem may make the decision obvious.
- Your client group may restrict your choice.
- You may work in a department, unit or area which already has a clear idea of the model or frame of reference it wishes to use.
- Your personal knowledge and expertise may be limited in the use of some approaches or techniques.
- Your own personal style may distinctly favour a particular approach.

If you do have the opportunity to choose, the latter two considerations are likely to be the most significant. The deciding questions are:

- Will this structure best meet my patient's needs?

- Can I use it effectively and be comfortable with it?

Once a decision has been taken, techniques must also be chosen. With some frames of reference the choices will have been made for you, but others give more freedom. There is nothing wrong in keeping the options open, or moving in and out of available techniques — so long as these do not conflict or render each other less effective.

Why are structures necessary?

Using a structure provides you with the mental equivalent of a map to guide the treatment process. It may also help to limit possibilities and to focus the mind in a particular direction. Correctly used, it will help you to make therapeutic decisions by offering a coherent framework for practice, relevant to the needs of the patient, and may aid multidisciplinary communication by clarifying expectations and the basis for therapy.

Choosing a structure is the equivalent of equipping yourself with a pair of spectacles with a specially tinted filter. Once you have put them on, your view of the world is coloured and some shades may be excluded. Another useful analogy is to think of structures as tools in a rack. If you need to knock-in a nail, you automatically pick a hammer, not a screwdriver — but to drill a hole you can choose from a hand drill, brace and bit, bradawl, auger, electric drill or pillar drill. This may seem confusing, but only if you are not a carpenter; if you are, the choice will be obvious. Similarly, the selection of a model or frame of reference becomes easier when you have expertise as a therapist.

Selection of a structure is contextual: it depends on your own skills, interests and concepts, the needs of your patient/client or the location in which you are working. It is, arguably, perfectly possible to be a good therapist without ever conciously using a model or frame of reference, provided that your core skills are well developed (but using one might make you even better). It is equally possible to know 'all that there is to be knowed' about models and frames of reference, and to remain an indifferent therapist. The tool is only as good as the skill and understanding of the person using it — and we all know that 'bad workmen blame their tools'.

It will also become clear that some approaches and techniques require much more experience or expertise than others — we all have to start somewhere, but it is not wise to attempt to use a technique which you only partially understand unless you have found someone experienced to give you close supervision until you become proficient.

Score code for questionnaire on p. 13

If you got a mix of letters, you are working eclectically, as many therapists do, or you might be using the problem solving model.

Mainly	a	—	you are working within the traditional rehabilitation model.
Several	b	—	you have strong humanist leanings (and/or you are working in the community).
	c	—	behavioural approach.
	d	—	developmental model and approaches.
	q	—	you have reacted to the current managerial changes in the NHS.
	e	—	educational model and techniques.
	f	—	problem solving model.
	g	—	psychodynamic model.
	a/r	—	rehabilitation with biomechanical approach.
	m	—	medical model.

This quiz should not, of course, be taken too seriously — there is absolutely nothing scientific about it. However, it does serve to illustrate that different structures have differing languages, utilize different techniques, and achieve differing aims. Start listening to your colleagues and see whether they give themselves away.

SUGGESTED READING

The following references will give you more information about terminology and the justification for, and development of, models and frames of reference. However, such discussion is detailed and often contradictory and it may be more comprehensible if you return to it when you have finished reading this study guide.

Creek J (ed) 1990 Occupational therapy and mental health; principles, skills and practice. Churchill Livingstone, Edinburgh (ch 1 History of the profession; ch 2 Knowledge base of OT; ch 3 Development of a paradigm)

Javetz, Katz 1989 Knowledgeability of theories of occupational therapy practitioners in Israel. American Journal of Occupational Therapy 43: 10

Hopkins H L, Smith H D (eds) 1988 Willard & Spackman's occupational therapy, 7th edn. Lippincott, Philadelphia (ch 3 Theory and philosophy)

Kielhofner G 1985 A Model of human occupations. Williams & Wilkins, Baltimore (Introduction)

Mosey A C 1981 Occupational therapy: configuration of a profession. Raven Press, New York (ch 4 Definition of a model; ch 12 Definition of frames of reference)

Mosey A C 1986 Psychosocial components of occupational therapy. Raven Press, New York (ch 1 the profession; ch 20 Frames of reference)

Reed K L 1984 Models of practice in occupational therapy. Williams & Wilkins, Baltimore (ch 1 Terminology; ch 2 Model building; ch 3 The use of models; ch 4 Characteristics and sources of a good model; ch 5 Metamodels)

Young M, Quinn E 1991 Theories and practice of occupational therapy. Churchill Livingstone, Edinburgh (ch 1 Terms and definitions; ch 2 Theoretical perspectives; ch 3 Frames of reference in OT)

2

Frames of reference

When using a frame of reference as a primary basis for treatment, the therapist begins from a distinct viewpoint which automatically includes or excludes a range of explanations about the patient, his needs and problems and the type of therapy he requires.

Each frame of reference stems from a distinct base of philosophy and theory. They do not, therefore, readily combine; indeed, they tend to contradict each other. That being said, the approaches and techniques which originate from each one are frequently used eclectically within the context of other models (e.g. rehabilitation, education, problem solving), and the general approaches of each frame of reference have been highly influential in the development of occupational therapy.

Included in this category are the following.

Physiological frame of reference

Behavioural frame of reference

Cognitive frame of reference

Psychodynamic frame of reference

Humanist frame of reference

THE PHYSIOLOGICAL FRAME OF REFERENCE

This frame of reference is based on a view of the individual as a biological organism whose behavi-

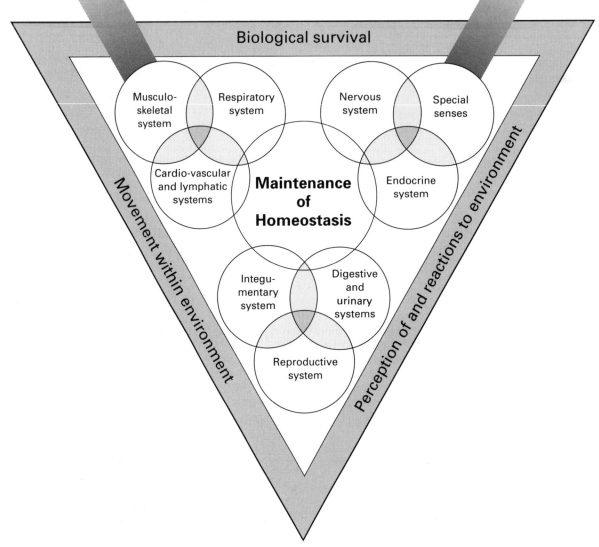

Fig. 2.1 The physiological frame of reference.

our depends on genetically determined factors, combined with the effective action of the nervous and endocrine systems and the ability of the body to maintain homeostasis (steady physiological state). Electrochemical neurological processes control behaviour and the individual's ability to respond to and learn from the environment. Performance depends on the integrity and interactions of all body systems, principally the musculoskeletal system, cardiovascular system, neurological system and the special senses.

Approaches

The physiological frame of reference has given rise to two distinct and contradictory approaches:

- the **biomechanical** approach;
- the **neurodevelopmental** approach.

Although both approaches are soundly based on physiology, each uses a distinct knowledge base, and the resultant techniques are mutually exclusive. Unless this is clearly understood, there is room for a good deal of confusion and consequently ineffective therapy. Practitioners who are old enough to remember the revolution in therapy which occurred during the early 1970s, when neurodevelopmental techniques began to take over from biomechanical ones in the treatment of brain damaged patients, will recall the frequent and acrimonious arguments between proponents of the opposing views. (A debate which has not entirely resolved even now.)

As a generalization, the biomechanical approach is reductionist in philosophy and is used in the rehabilitation of musculoskeletal or peripheral neurological injury, whilst the neurodevelopmental approach is more holistic in nature and is used in the treatment of trauma or developmental delay/ regression affecting the sensori-motor systems in children or adults.

The most significant opposing principles of the two approaches are summarized in Table 2, although application will vary in accordance with the needs of individuals with specific conditions.

THE BIOMECHANICAL APPROACH

This approach is based on *kinesiology*, which combines neuromuscular physiology, musculoskeletal anatomy and biomechanics. It uses the laws of mechanics, e.g. leverage, gravity, friction and resistance, to improve function or solve a performance problem. Physical exercise — isotonic, isometric and isokinetic (although the latter is not applicable in OT) — is used to increase the strength and bulk of muscles, and to improve stamina and work tolerance. Exercise is also used to increase or restore the range of movement at a joint. In a typical training or retraining programme, the individual is required to work as close to his functional limits as possible, without undue fatigue, in order to gain improvement. The performance 'goal posts' are continually moved as improvement occurs. Grading of the elements in the exercise programme, e.g. assistance, resist-

Table 2 Comparison of neurodevelopmental approach and biomechanical approach

Neurodevelopmental approach	Biomechanical approach
Work first for control and pattern of gross movements	Work first for functional use; may promote fine movements
Always work from proximal to distal	May work from distal to proximal
In the upper limb, use extensor/abductor patterns; promote grip last; avoid stimulation of flexor surfaces	In the upper limb, work for flexion and functional use — promote grip early; may use stimulation of flexor surfaces
In the lower limb, work against extensor thrust and adductor patterns	In the lower limb, promote knee and hip extension and stability of knee and ankle
Delay walking and standing until developmentally ready	Stand/walk as early as possible
Grade therapy according to developmental stages: work within limits of current level until ability to progress is established	Grade therapy according to progress: work at or just beyond limits of current capacity
Use orthoses and external supports with discretion and as a last resort	Use orthoses as routine
Emphasize treatment of whole body to achieve symmetry	Emphasize treatment of affected part
Emphasize sensory integration and proprioception	Emphasize functional and protective sensation

ance, range, speed, duration and repetition, is a crucial part of the therapist's role.

Biomechanically based OT, in which the performance of an activity is used to produce specific movements, and where the elements in the performance must be precisely controlled and graded, requires an imaginative and ingenious attitude on the part of the therapist. The use of such activities involves thought and preparation and, unless correctly used and monitored, can be ineffective. It is almost inevitable that patient choice in the selection of an activity will be limited by the constraints of meeting specific objectives. Even so, such therapy has been criticised as insufficiently precise, and this, together with the reaction against 'craft-work' and the desire to appear technologically advanced, has resulted in the use of somewhat stereotyped non-productive activities as exercises — a trend which was very noticeable during the mid 1970s, but which is now decreasing. (It is my own view that patients whose needs are better met by exercise than activity, or who actually prefer exercise, should be referred to a physiotherapist).

There is currently a renewed interest in the specific remedial use of activities as it is appreciated that the combined psychological and physical benefits of constructive, practical or creative activities may outweigh the disadvantages of any lack of precision in physical application. Recently, some interesting adaptations for computers have been produced, together with equipment which uses surface electrodes to translate specific muscle contractions into the switching of electric apparatus. This is sometimes used in conjunction with biofeedback techniques. Thorough physical assessment and measurement of function is an essential precursor to therapy, and should be repeated at frequent intervals in order to monitor progress and upgrade treatment.

The accelerated pace of recovery from trauma due to improved medical and surgical techniques during the past two decades has rendered rehabilitation unnecesary in some cases and has generally resulted in much shorter hospitalization, which has left little time for graded activity programmes to be implemented. Biomechanical techniques are therefore mainly used to treat individuals with more serious injuries or conditions requiring longer-term treatment, which is often undertaken on an out-patient basis.

The scientific aspect of biomechanics — the application of mechanical principles to the analysis of human movement or the design of aids, orthoses or prostheses — is primarily of use to the occupational therapist in designing aids to daily living or therapeutic adaptations to remedial apparatus. It is also useful in research.

Q Where do you stand on the question of the use of activities for specific physical treatment? To what extent should activities be adapted? Is adaptation effective? Is it too time-consuming? Should occupational therapists use non-productive 'activities'? How do patients react to this form of therapy? Discuss these points with some colleagues: you may well get a wide range of firmly held opinions.

Summary of the biomechanical approach

Metamodel: Reductionist.

Origin of problem: An illness, injury or congenital disorder has affected the strength, range or coordination of bodily movement, with consequent limitation of normal function for the individual.

Primary assumptions:
- The application of a graded programme of exercise based on kinesiological principles will restore normal or near normal function.
- Biomechanical principles can be used to provide aids, orthoses or adaptive equipment to overcome residual disability.

Terminology: Patient; therapist; disability; function.

Patient/therapist relationship: The therapist prescribes, directs and advises; the patient actively cooperates.

Examples of application: Hand injuries; fractures; peripheral nerve lesions; amputees; burns; cardiac conditions.

Examples of techniques: Graded physical treatment, e.g. to promote muscle power, joint range, endurance. Adapted activities — craft, technical, games.

Adapted apparatus — e.g. cycles, lathes, pulleys, springs, special handles.

Adapted equipment for activities of daily living.

Assessment for, and provision of, wheelchairs and adapted vehicles.

Provision of, and training in use of orthoses, prostheses.

Some forms of biofeedback.

Criteria for evaluation of outcome: The patient will show measurable improvement in physical function.

Advantages: Biomechanical techniques are well researched and can be shown to produce improvement in physical function. Because improving functional ability is the chief goal and results are relatively rapid, the patient can see positive benefits as treatment progresses and is motivated to continue. Residual disabilities can be overcome by aids and orthoses.

Disadvantages: Because treatment has to be very specific to produce results, patient choice in the selection of activities may be restricted; there is a danger that the programmes may become stereotyped. Activity programmes take time to set up and prepare and are impractical where treatment time is limited. An overly physical bias may result in wider social, environmental or psychological problems being ignored.

SUGGESTED READING

The references given below are quite specific, but you will also find relevant material in the references quoted for the rehabilitation model.

Galley P M, Forster A L 1987 Human movement, 2nd edn. Churchill Livingstone, Edinburgh (Basic review of anatomy, movement mechanics and principles of exercise for physiotherapy students.)
Mills D, Fraser C 1989 Therapeutic activities for the upper limb. Winslow Press, Bicester

Norkin C, White J 1985 Measurement of joint motion. F A Davis, Philadelphia
Pedretti L (ed) 1985 Occupational therapy: practice skills for physical dysfunction, 2nd edn. C V Mosby, St. Louis (chs 5, 6, 7, 8, 9, 18)
Trombley C A 1983 Occupational therapy for physical dysfunction, 2nd edn. Williams & Wilkins, Baltimore (chs 7, 8)

THE NEURODEVELOPMENTAL APPROACH

I have used this term to encompass a number of distinct but related approaches and techniques which you will find referred to as separate models in some books. They share the common link of being based on principles of neuromuscular facilitation and sensory integration, and of having a strongly developmental base. Variations have evolved for use in the treatment of physical disorders, psychiatric disorders and mental handicap.

In physical contexts, the emphasis is on a sequence of interventions and the use of sensory and perceptual input and voluntary or reflex output. The aim is to promote the attainment of, and progression through, stages of increasing skill and complexity, to a point where potential has been developed to the maximum possible for the individual.

In the treatment of psychiatric disorders or mental handicap, the emphasis is on the capacity of the individual to perceive and react correctly to people and the environment. Recognizing the strong link between sensory input and motor output, the therapist may use sensori-motor activity to stimulate perception and priorioception, thus raising the general level of activity where this is retarded.

Typically, the primary techniques associated with this approach were evolved by physiotherapists, and in unadapted form are not readily related to activity based occupational therapy, being more commonly used as an adjunct to it or precursor of it. However it is possible to adapt positioning for use in functional activity, and to incorporate basic neurodevelopmental principles into an activity based OT programme. Since the techniques are important ones for the therapist, they are summarized in more detail below.

Summary of the neurodevelopmental approach

Metamodel: Although many techniques are very precisely directed, developmentally one must regard an individual as an integrated, reactive person in whom a deficit in one area will affect the whole. This approach is therefore organismic in general outlook, although it may become reductionist in application.

Origin of problem: The adult or child shows developmental delay or regression to a primitive neurodevelopmental level, due to congenital or acquired damage to the brain, genetic abnormality or the effects of other illness or injury.

Primary assumptions:

- Neurological development occurs in stages: these stages relate to the acquisition of sensori-motor skills. Stages cannot be 'jumped' or missed. In order to gain or regain function, the individual must be taken through a normal developmental sequence.
- There is a strong link between sensory input and motor output.
- Use of proprioception, positioning and reflexes can facilitate normal movement, posture and reactions.

Terminology: Therapist; patient/client; therapy. (The language of the specific neurodevelopmental technique is employed.)

Patient/therapist relationship: The therapist assesses and decides on the intervention; the patient cooperates, actively or passively.

Examples of applications:

Children: spasticity; 'clumsy child'; brain damage; mental handicap; dystrophy.

Adults: Learning difficulties (mental handicap); physical conditions, e.g. cerebral vascular accident, head injury, multiple sclerosis, motor neurone disease, parkinsonism, spinal cord

lesions; psychiatric disorders, e.g. schizophrenia, institutionalization, dementia.

Techniques used:

Bobath technique: A bilateral approach to the treatment of hemiplegia or spasticity utilizing positioning, weight bearing, reflex inhibition and sensory facilitation. This can be adapted for use with OT activities more readily than some other techniques (Bobath 1986).

Basic principles include:

- Positioning the patient in a manner which will inhibit the development of abnormal reflexes and synergies and reduce abnormal muscle tone, enabling the patient to re-learn normal movement patterns.
- Facilitating correct movement by positioning, correct handling, use of sensory stimulation and the use of key control points on the body.
- Working through a developmental sequence — lying, 'all-fours', trunk control, sitting, standing, weight transfer, stepping, walking.
- Involving both sides of the body in all activities. Use of activities which *promote*: crossing the midline with arm; diagonal patterns of arm use; special bilateral grip; weight bearing through affected side; trunk rotation; and which *avoid*: flexor patterns in the upper limb and extensor patterns in the lower limb; stimulation of associated reactions.

Proprioceptive neuromuscular facilitation (PNF): A technique which uses positioning and patterns of movement in developmental sequence and emphasizes sensory input, visual cues and verbal commands to produce maximum input. Sensory input stimulates and facilitates motor output.

Sensory integration: This stresses the importance of the integration and interpretation of all sensory inputs, and the necessity of promoting integrated sensory stimulation to develop or restore function. Activity using touch, vibration, sound, smell and colour is geared to stimulation at subcortical level, with particular attention to vestibular and proprioceptive input. This technique was developed by Ayres (1972) for use with children and neurologically damaged adults. Another version of the technique has been used in a psychiatric setting following the work of King (1974) with schizophrenics; she advocated the use of activities which increase and promote vestibular stimulation, bilateral integration and the integration of primitive postural reflexes to overcome synaptic barriers and promote normal body image, posture, righting reactions and reflexes.

Rood technique: This uses similar principles to sensory integration and PNF but emphasizes tactile stimulation (brushing, icing, tapping, pressure and stretch reflexes). Rood is both an OT and a physiotherapist but the technique is more related to PT than OT.

Conductive education (Peto): A highly structured and formal system mainly used with children (although some work has been done with adults) based on a planned, intensive, programme aimed at achieving goals for each individual. The work employs a blend of cognitive and neuro-developmental principles. The therapist acts as a 'conductor,' planning tasks, facilitating movement, using formalized verbalization to assist actions; the patient also says what he is doing at each stage as he does it. Personal control and responsibility are emphasized; rhythm is used to promote and initiate movement. Conductive education is currently attracting considerable interest, but it is not yet widely used by British OTs. Some therapists have incorporated the concept of patient verbalization as an adjunct to other therapy.

Criteria for evaluation of outcome: The individual has achieved improvement in sensori-motor function and/or has achieved the normal patterns of movement responses and abilities for his or her age/sex.

Advantages: When used correctly and intensively, these therapies produce good results, particularly in preventing the development of abnormal patterns of movement and deformity following neurological damage.

Disadvantages: Unless used intensively, skilfully and correctly by all members of the treatment team, results are likely to be disappointing. Special training is required to use most techniques effectively. Working neurodevelopmentally is time consuming and functional recovery in the brain damaged adult, e.g. walking, may be delayed with consequent frustration for the patient. The techniques are less suitable for use with very elderly patients. Although vigorously promoted by enthusiasts, there is some recent criticism of the physiological assumptions on which therapy is based; studies are difficult to compare and evaluate, and it has been argued that good results are due more to the intensive nature of the treatment and the excellent rapport which develops between the patient and an expert practitioner, than to the techniques themselves. Extreme, highly intensive, versions of some techniques, particularly as applied to children, are still very controversial.

SUGGESTED READING

Bobath B 1986 Adult hemiplegia: evaluation and treatment, 2nd edn. Heinemann, London

Cotton E, Kinsman R 1983 Conductive education for adult hemiplegia. Churchill Livingstone, Edinburgh

Creek J (ed) 1990 Occupational therapy and mental health; principles, skills and practice. Churchill Livingstone, Edinburgh (ch 11 Sensory integration)

Eggers O 1988 Occupational therapy in the rehabilitation of adult hemiplegia. Heinemann, London

Finlay L 1988 Occupational therapy practice in psychiatry. Croom Helm, London (ch 2 Ayers)

Macdonald J 1990 The international course on conductive education at the Peto Andras State Institute for Conductive Education, Budapest. British Journal of Occupational Therapy. 53 (7) 295–300

Mosey A C 1986 Psychosocial components of occupational therapy. Raven Press, New York (ch 31 Sensory integration)

Pedretti L (ed) 1985 Occupational therapy: practice skills for physical dysfunction, 2nd edn. C V Mosby, St Louis (ch 8 Evaluation of reflexes; ch 9 Evaluation of sensation, perception, cognition; ch 13 Neurophysiology of sensori-motor approaches; ch 14 Rood; ch 15 Brunnstrom; ch 16 Bobath; ch 17 PNF)

Ross M, Burdick D 1981 Sensory integration. Slack, New Jersey

Trombley C A 1983 Occupational therapy for physical dysfunction, 2nd edn. Williams & Wilkins, Baltimore (ch 6 Rood; Bobath; PNF)

Wilcock A A 1986 Occupational therapy approaches to stroke. Churchill Livingstone, Edinburgh

Zolton B, Seiv E, Freishtat B 1986 Perceptual and cognitive dysfunction in the adult stroke patient, 2nd edn. Slack, New Jersey

Note: These references deal primarily with application to adults. For use of techniques with children, you will need to refer to specialized literature.

THE BEHAVIOURAL FRAME OF REFERENCE

Behaviourism is primarily a theory of learning. It has developed from the original research into stimulus response learning by Pavlov, Thorndike and Watson, followed by the work on *operant conditioning* by Skinner and many others. Research has concentrated on proposing explanations of observable animal and human behaviours in terms of interactions with the environment. The environment provides stimuli to which the individual responds. The individual is able to appreciate the outcome of the response by means of feedback. Responses which are rewarded or are useful to the individual in satisfying drives are continued and become part of the behavioural repertoire. Those which are unsuccessful, or which achieve unpleasant results, are discontinued.

Strict behaviourists believe that man has little

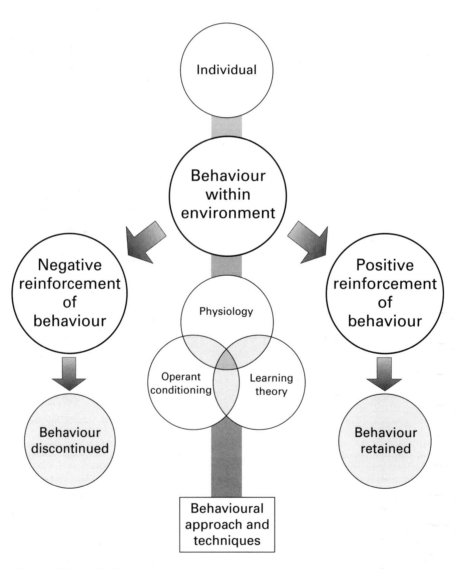

Fig. 2.2 The behavioural frame of reference.

choice in deciding how to behave — he is instead programmed to react through conditioning derived from past experience. Purists in this field discount all interior motivators, such as emotions and thoughts, either as products of behaviour, or as internal, unobservable events which cannot be studied objectively.

Bandura extended the concept of operant conditioning and recognized that the individual does not need to experience the reinforcement personally, but may learn by observing the results of the behaviour of others — a process called *modelling*, which has important implications for therapy.

Other researchers have moved away from the extreme behaviourist position held by Skinner, and have tended to include some elements of cognitive theory, particularly aspects of the information processing theories of memory. This has produced a pragmatic, structured approach to teaching and learning which is very relevant to the therapist.

Few occupational therapists apply the behavioural frame of reference in strict and unadapted form, but behavioural theories have been influential in both education and therapy, and are used in behavioural modification and desensitization programmes, and in skill training and programmed learning. A feature of all such programmes is the breaking down of tasks into simple component parts and sequences and the use of very clear statements of objectives, goals and methods of instruction. Schedules of reinforcement, designed to meet the learning needs of the individual, are also important.

Summary of the behavioural approach

Metamodel: Reductionist.

Origin of problem: The individual has acquired (through faulty learning due to inappropriate reinforcement and/or environment) an 'undesirable' (inappropriate, damaging, unproductive) behaviour, or failed to acquire a 'desirable' (appropriate, utilitarian) one.

Primary assumptions

- An individual can only be studied in terms of his observable behaviour.

- All actions performed by the individual are regarded as behaviour; this includes language.
- Behaviour occurs in response to stimuli, which promote or decrease it.
- All behaviour is learnt. Behaviour can be unlearnt (extinguished) as well as learnt.
- Learning occurs in response to reinforcement, which is either provided extrinsically by the environment or intrinsically by the behaviour.
- Intermittent schedules of reinforcement are the most effective.
- A positive reinforcer must be carefully selected to be appropriate to the individual and must be correctly and consistently used.
- Behaviour can be reduced to a simple sequence of responses: these can be taught separately if required, or chained in sequence. Complex sequences combine to produce 'molar behaviour' — the response of the whole organism.
- Learning programmes should be designed to meet the exact requirements of the individual.

Terminology: Behaviourism has a distinct language, which must be acquired by the therapist if he or she is to work comfortably within the approach. Frequently used terms include: patient (client); therapist; classical conditioning; operant conditioning; stimulus-response (SR) conditioning; deconditioning; extinction; positive/negative reinforcement; schedules of reinforcment; reward/punishment; time out; modelling; shaping; cueing; training; behavioural contract; behaviour modification; goal planning; behavioural objectives.

Patient/therapist relationship: In the strict form of behaviourism, the patient has little to do with goal setting and need not even be capable of cooperation since the therapist controls all elements of the situation. In the more usual (modified) form, the patient and therapist may agree a behavioural contract, or the patient may participate in goal setting.

Examples of applications: Learning difficulties (mental handicap); skill deficits; brain injuries;

psychiatric disorders, e.g. phobias, anxiety states; dependency related problems, e.g. substance abuse; behavioural problems/challenging behaviours; institutionalization.

Examples of techniques

Behaviour modification: The basic principles of this technique are usually adapted for use in OT programmes. The technique can be used both to teach a desirable behaviour or to remove an undesirable one.

A typical behaviour modification programme might involve:

- Setting a precise behavioural objective for the patient to achieve.
- Deciding on a positive reinforcer or reward to be used following successful performance, e.g. food or drink; an enjoyable activity; praise; affection; a privilege. (At this point a behavioural contract specifying both the desired behaviour and the reward may be drawn up between patient and therapist.)
- Providing opportunities for the behaviour to occur; prompting, shaping and cueing the behaviour if necessary.
- Consistently providing the reward when the behaviour (or, at first, a close approximation to it) is achieved.
- Gradually withdrawing or reducing the frequency of the reward once the behaviour has become an established part of the repertoire.

Other techniques which may be used include: social modelling; token economy; desensitization of phobias; programmed learning; chaining and backward chaining; room management techniques; biofeedback.

Criteria for evaluation of outcome: A previously specified behavioural performance has been observed to be consistently achieved. (Or an undesirable behaviour has been eliminated from the repertoire.)

Advantages: Precise objectives are set, and achievement of objectives is measurable in performance terms. The associated techniques are of particular use for individuals who have moderate or severe learning difficulties, challenging behaviours or behavioural disturbances, and for

WRITING BEHAVIOURAL OBJECTIVES

Writing clear behavioural objectives is an essential therapeutic skill which is often used, even when not employing a strictly behavioural approach. It is also a skill which can be carried out with insufficient precision. As proficiency is mainly a matter of practice, you may find the following exercise helpful.

An objective must contain both the specification of the performance and criteria by which successful completion can be measured. It is usually formed as follows:

- **Person** (student/client)
- **Precise performance** (defines what is to be done)
- **Conditions** (indicates when, where, how often, how long, with/without specified form of help, etc.)

e.g. The student [*person*] will point to the carpal bones on the skeleton and will correctly name each one [*precise performance*] at the first attempt and without reference to notes [*conditions*].

If you would like to practise writing behavioural objectives, try producing some for this client:

Jenny is a 16 year old girl with severe learning difficulties. She has been referred with the aim of 'improving her independence in feeding'. When you visit her at lunch time, you observe that initially, she makes no attempt to feed herself. She is able to grasp a spoon when it is placed in her hand and rather messily tries to get some food onto it. Once she has the food in her mouth, she immediately tries to get some more onto the spoon and into her mouth without leaving time for chewing and swallowing. Consequently, she spits out food or chokes and becomes very frustrated. She abandons her attempts at eating after a few minutes.

1 Write some clear behavioural objectives for the first stage of your treatment.
2 Which aspect would you tackle first? Would you work towards this in stages? If so, how might you write specific objectives for this?

people with fears originating from situational conditioning. Learning does not have to depend on patient motivation or cooperation. Teaching can be tailored to individual needs. Specific skills and sub-skills can be learnt in small stages. Behaviours can be unlearnt.

Disadvantages: Although basic behavioural theory is often used, effective application of behavioural techniques is time consuming and must be implemented with great precision and expertise by all concerned; this normally requires additional training for therapists. Incorrectly applied behaviour modification is at best useless and at worst damaging. Each objective must be very carefully phrased, specifying the behaviour and the conditions under which it will be performed: if this is done 'fuzzily', therapy may be ineffective and measurement of success of dubious validity. Learning may not generalize and may fade once the reinforcement is withdrawn. The reductionist approach ignores emotional and cognitive explanations of behaviour. An overly strict application of positive/negative reinforcement, particularly if there is any element of punishment, carries ethical implications, and unpleasant echoes of Orwell's *1984*.

SUGGESTED READING

Any psychology textbook will contain basic behavioural theory. The books listed under the education model also give good summaries of theory. Books on therapy for mentally handicapped or brain damaged individuals frequently contain information on the use of behavioural techniques.

Bandura A 1977 Social learning theory. Prentice Hall, New Jersey
Bigge M 1987 Learning theories for teachers, 4th edn. Harper & Row, New York
Bruce M A & Borg B 1987 Frames of reference in psychiatric occupational therapy. Slack, New Jersey (The behavioural frame of reference)
Gagné R M 1977 The conditions of learning and theory of instruction, 3rd edn. Holt Saunders, Eastbourne

Jones M C 1983 Behaviour problems in handicapped children. Souvenir Press, London
Lovell R B 1987 Adult learning. Croom Helm, London
Mosey A C 1981 Occupational therapy: configuration of a profession. Raven Press, New York (ch 14 The acquisitional frame of reference)
Mosey A C 1986 Psychosocial components of occupational therapy. Raven Press, New York (ch 25 & ch 26 The acquisitional frame of reference)
Reed K L 1984 Models of practice in occupational therapy. Williams & Wilkins, Baltimore (ch 6 Supermodels)
Yule W & Carr J Behaviour modification for the mentally handicapped. Croom Helm, London
Willson M 1987 Occupational therapy in long-term psychiatry, 2nd edn. Churchill Livingstone, Edinburgh (ch 1 Behavioural models)

THE COGNITIVE FRAME OF REFERENCE

In direct contrast to the behaviourists, cognitive psychologists are primarily concerned with phenomena, i.e. subjective experiences. They seek to understand the processes of the mind, such as perception, memory and conceptualization, and to provide theories about how the individual forms relationships between concepts, interprets structures and makes sense of the environment. Links are made between the effectiveness with which the individual manages these processes and his ability to learn and develop rules, skills and roles, and also to plan and carry out appropriate behaviour.

An understanding of such cognitive theories is essential if the therapist is to assess and identify the individual's difficulties in perception, memory and learning, and therefore to construct more effective ways of presenting information or improving cognitive skills.

The cognitive frame of reference has evolved different approaches and techniques, which some may consider to be models in their own right, combining the physiology of cognition, elements of learning theory and elements of developmental or humanistic theories in various proportions.

Gestalt psychology (Wertheimer et al) is concerned with the investigation of perception and the formulation of laws which govern how we perceive the world as a whole. (This should not be confused with *gestalt therapy* which, although influenced by the ideas of gestalt psychology — such as perception of patterns and wholes, or desire for closure — deals with the whole person, not merely the

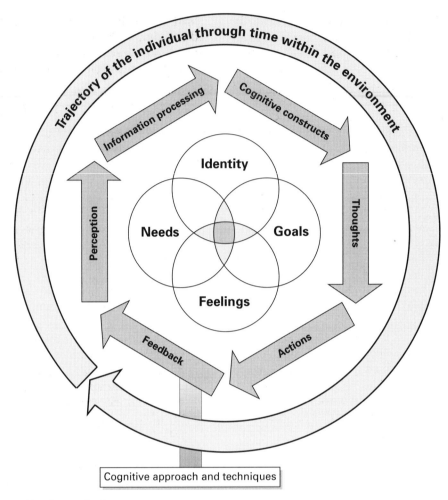

Fig. 2.3 The cognitive frame of reference.

organizational rules of perception. This is better viewed as a humanistic psychotherapy.)

Early cognitive research was mainly linked with neurophysiology and this aspect continues. Some researchers use sophisticated technology to investigate the physiological changes which occur in the brain as a result of perceiving or learning, and attempt to identify which parts of the brain are responsible for specific cognitive functions. Despite this research, at great deal is still unknown about the nature of thought and the means whereby information is actually stored and processed.

Cognitivists working in educational psychology

seem to be more concerned with explaining the processes by which ideas are formed in the mind than investigating neurochemical actions. Other cognitive psychologists seek to use their theories and models of mental processes to enable them to predict how an individual is likely to behave in a given situation. They see the ability of the individual to learn insightfully, to problem solve, to use his past experiences and to plan his future actions as important. The individual's internal constructs of past, present, and particularly the future, are of significance.

In cognitive field theory (Lewin), a complex topological explanation is proposed of how each individual possesses a life space which continually changes, and in which directional currents propel or repel him as he seeks to travel towards personal goals.

Cognitive approaches to the treatment of psychiatric illness or personality disorder have been developed, some of which are described in the section on humanism (p. 35) since they seem more appropriately linked to psychotherapy. For example, Ellis used cognitive approaches in the treatment of mental disorder, arguing that disorders are due to faulty ways of thinking about the world and the misinterpretation of information. He introduced *rational emotive therapy*, summarized by the 'ABC theory': **A** — Antecedant: a fact, event, behaviour or attitude which, **B** — influences the patient's Belief which, **C** — decides the Consequence. He also coined the expression '*muster*batory behaviour' to describe acts originating from irrational compulsive belief patterns.

Beck developed *cognitive therapy*, a less directive and interpretive style, based on helping the client to analyse the interactions of his thoughts, emotions and behaviours. Other workers look for 'life themes' — persistant rules or attitudes which predominate in and direct the client's behaviour.

Cognitive-behavioural approaches are highly structured and rely on methods which seek to change the content of thought — particularly anxious, depressive or obsessive thought patterns — thereby improving affect and behaviour. Other approaches use the theory of social modelling, or techniques of behavioural rehearsal or role play.

In occupational therapy a variety of cognitive approaches have been developed. Some techniques are used with brain-injured individuals, and these use assessments of perception, sequencing, logic, memory or constructional sensori-motor function (Cotnab, Rivermead). Techniques such as *reality orientation* and *reminiscence therapy* are primarily cognitive. For psychiatric disorders, Allen (1985) has evolved a structured developmental/cognitive approach in which activities are presented in a manner and at a level applicable to the participant's cognitive abilities. Llorens (1986) proposes a sensory processing model for activity analysis which links cognitive and sensory integrative approaches.

With such a diversity of theoretical backgrounds and techniques, this is not an easy frame of reference to summarize and the description of the approach is necessarily highly generalized.

Summary of the cognitive approach

Metamodel: Organismic. Thoughts, mental processes, emotions and behaviour are closely linked.

Origin of problem: Faulty learning, incorrect or incomplete cognitive processing, incorrect interpretation or distortion of perceptions, compulsive or irrational thought processes, failure to establish an autonomous identity or to develop a positive self-concept, and general misinterpretations of reality produce dysfunctions in social interactions, emotional control, cognitive strategies or ability to perform activities.

Primary assumptions:

* Cognition is a complex process which may be explained by various theories.
* Each individual has a unique experience and interpretation of his environment.
* Behaviour and emotions originate with thoughts: thoughts are influenced by perceptions of past and future events.
* Perceptions of self, and the way in which the individual views his past actions or plans future ones are also governed by cognitive processes.
* Dysfunctional individuals can be helped to become functional by an analysis of cognitive processes, by improving knowledge and learning strategies and by teaching 'healthy', positive and effective cognitive strategies to replace 'unhealthy', negative or ineffective ones.

Terminology: Patient; client; therapist (and the language of particular techniques).

Patient/therapist relationship: This depends on the technique being used; it may be analytical, directive or facilitatory.

Examples of applications: Physical conditions, e.g. brain injury, cerebral vascular accident; mental handicap; psychiatric disorders, e.g. anxiety, depression, obsessional states, phobias, dementia.

Examples of techniques

Physical: Perceptual training; conceptual training; memory training; therapy for agnosias/apraxias.

Psychiatric/behavioural: Social modelling; behavioural rehearsal; cognitive modelling; scripting; role play; assertiveness training; 'homework' — e.g. diary, cognitive tasks; relaxation techniques; stress management; reminiscence; reality orientation; problem solving training.

Criteria for evaluation of outcome: The individual reports and/or the therapist observes improvement in perceptual or cognitive skills leading to positive changes in performance and/or affect.

Advantages: In psychiatry, cognitive techniques generally offer practical strategies which involve the patient in identifying the elements of his feelings/thoughts/behaviours which he wants to change, and then taking action to achieve this. This is reported to produce quite rapid, observable, positive results. Interpretations of the 'unconscious' causation of behaviour are avoided and therapy may therefore be more acceptable to the patient. Cognitive developmental approaches can be helpful where patients are cognitively regressed or brain-damaged (Allen 1985). Perceptual training is widely used in the treatment of cerebral vascular accidents and brain injury.

Disadvantages: Some of the theoretical models or explanations of cognitive function are very complex; some techniques are based on hypotheses which are still not well researched and cannot be 'proved' since they deal with subjective material. A great deal concerning the processes of cognition is still conjectural. Some models require that the patient is of 'normal' intelligence for therapy to be effective.

SUGGESTED READING

Most psychology textbooks contain chapters on cognitive processes.

Allen C K 1985 Occupational therapy for psychiatric disorders: measurement and management of cognitive disabilities. Little, Brown & Co. Inc., Boston

Bandura A 1977 Social learning theory. Prentice Hall, New Jersey

Beck A T 1976 Cognitive therapy and the emotional disorders. Meridian, New York

Creek J 1990 Occupational therapy and mental health: principles, skills and practice. Churchill Livingstone, Edinburgh (ch 12 Cognitive approaches)

Bigge M 1987 Learning theories for teachers, 4th edn. Harper & Row, New York (chs 8, 9, 14 — description of cognitive field psychology)

Bruce M A & Borg B 1987 Frames of reference in psychiatric occupational therapy. Slack, New Jersey (Cognitive frame of reference; cognitive-behavioural frame of reference)

Pedretti L (ed) Occupational therapy: practice skills for physical dysfunction, 2nd edn. Mosby, St Louis (ch 9 Evaluation of perception and cognition)

Rimmer L 1982 Reality orientation: principles and practice. Winslow Press, Bicester

Zoltan B, Seiv E , Frieshtat B 1986 Perceptual and cognitive dysfunction in the adult stroke patient, 2nd edn. Slack, New Jersey

THE PSYCHODYNAMIC FRAME OF REFERENCE

The term *psychodynamic* has been chosen as an umbrella term to include the different, but related, theories which are concerned with the origins of an individual's personality and motivation, and with methods of helping the individual to gain insight and to achieve personal growth.

Occupational therapists in psychiatric practice frequently use a synthesis of techniques rather than one derived from a single school of psychoanalysis or psychotherapy. OT's do not, and should not, act as psychoanalysts, or as psychotherapists (unless having an additional qualification).

The psychodynamic frame of reference is unique in dealing with the unconscious motiv-

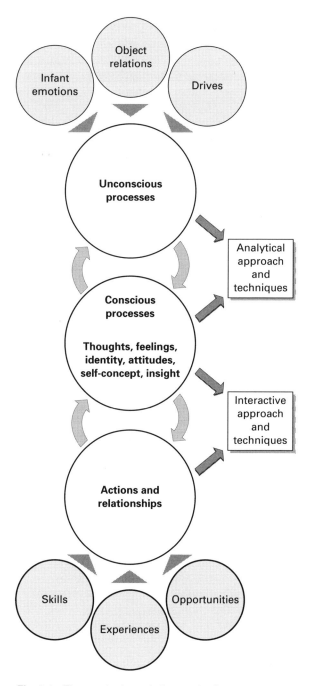

Fig. 2.4 The psychodynamic frame of reference.

ations for actions, interactions and beliefs, and the symbolic content of images and perceptions. Explanations for the unconscious basis of behav-iour differ, and include psychoanalytical theory, object relations theory, group theory, psychotherapy theories, and some elements of cognitive and developmental psychology and learning theory.

This is an area where theorists abound and generalizations are difficult. Two distinct approaches will be described:

1 The *analytical approach* — derived from psychoanalytical and object relations theories;
2 The *interactive approach* – derived from group theory and psychotherapy.

THE ANALYTICAL APPROACH

The classical form of psychoanalysis is that originated by Freud at the beginning of the 20th century. He created the terms which have passed into the language of analysis, e.g. *unconscious, preconscious, id, ego, superego* and *libido,* and proposed that the gratification of drives, especially sexuality, was the basis of human behaviour. According to Freudian theory, the development of the individual during infancy and childhood follows a series of stages. Fixation at, or regression to one of these early stages limits the development of an integrated personality.

Subsequently other schools of psychoanalysis have developed extending or deviating from Freud's original explanations of the basis of human personality. The most significant of these considers *object relations* — the perceptions of, and relationships with, people or desired objects, particularly those developed as a baby. These are considered to have a fundamental influence on subsequent relationships and behaviour.

Psychoanalysts share a deterministic view of the individual as motivated by unconscious or dimly perceived drives and emotions which direct behaviour and which are not subject to voluntary control ('push motivation'). Some of these unconscious forces are innate, others arise through the interpretation of past experiences, usually those gained by the very young child. The individual can, by a long process of analysis (during which the relationship with the analyst is a significant part of therapy), come to a better, but never complete, understanding of the reasons for his feelings and behaviour. This may help the individual to live a more satisfying and less anxious life. The analytical approach therefore takes a primarily retrospective view of human actions.

Since Freud, many theorists have developed their own ideas, following one or other of the above styles, or attempting a synthesis. The role of the analyst varies from the neutral to the directive and from the reflective to the actively interpretive or interactive. There are far too many notable names to mention them all, but some people who have produced innovatory and influential theories between the World Wars include:

- Freud (stages of sexuality; gratification of drives)
- Adler (will to power)
- Jung (dreams and symbols; archetypes and the collective unconscious)
- Klein (object relations; infantile experiences)
- Sullivan (object relations; juvenile anxiety)
- Winnicott (child/mother relationship)
- Guntrip (repressed ego)

Later theorists are even more numerous and the student is advised to read texts selectively to avoid becoming confused by elaborate and contradictory concepts.

The occupational therapist typically uses creative and projective techniques when using this approach, working with people as individuals or as a collection of individuals within a group. Analytical theories are concerned with the reasons for an individual's reactions to his own feelings or to other individuals or objects, not with his reactions to people in general or a group as a whole. The degree to which an occupational therapist may interpret the use of images and symbols by the patient, and the manner in which the therapist facilitates self-discovery, depends on the theory within which he is working, and the techniques with which he is familiar. Because of the highly potent nature of unconscious material, all such techniques should be used with discretion, following suitable training, and the practitioner must have access to adequate personal supervision. (The supervisor must be a person suitably qualified both to over-see the therapist's treatment of patients and also to deal with the dynamics of the

therapist's own needs, dilemmas and personal growth).

Summary of the analytical approach

Metamodel: Reductionist, based on the premise that a person is not capable of rational choices, behaviour being determined by unconscious drives and past experiences and feelings, which may be analysed to provide explanations of current behaviour and emotions.

Origin of problem: A deficit in or lack of integration of the personality, stemming from unconscious causes. The problem is usually described within the language of a particular theory. Examples: an unresolved conflict; fixation in or regression to an early developmental stage; lack of insight; failure to acknowledge sexuality; faulty early relationship with a parent.

Primary assumptions

(This summary deals with broad principles shared by the main schools of analysis, as interpreted in the context of OT. In analytical practice, there are marked differences between theorists which are reflected in the use of language and techniques.)

- Behaviour is governed by unconscious, irrational processes, linked to the gratification of basic drives.
- Early life, during which a person develops through psychosexual stages or stages in the development of relationships with persons and objects, has a lasting effect on personality.
- Conflicts, anxiety, guilt, depression or problems with relationships in later life are symptoms of unresolved unconscious conflicts originating in repressed memories of infancy and childhood.
- Subconscious material may surface in the form of dreams and symbols which may affect perceptions of reality.
- It is possible, through a lengthy process of analysis, to uncover the origins of symptoms, to bring material out of the unconscious, to gain insight, and thereby to resolve conflicts, anxieties and unsatisfactory relationships.

Terminology: Patient/client; analysand; therapist;

analyst; therapy; analysis, (. . . and the language of the particular theorist, e.g. Freud — ego, superego, libido, transference, counter-transference, projection, repression, unconscious, preconscious.)

Patient/therapist relationship: It is anticipated that a complex relationship occurs during an extended process of analysis, which involves mechanisms such as projection, transference and counter-transference. Although the occupational therapist is not functioning as a analyst, such relationships may develop and the therapist must be aware of his own mechanisms of defence or transference. The patient may develop some dependency on the therapist.

Examples of conditions treated: Anxiety states; affective disorders; sexual dysfunction; failure to develop a positive self-image; feelings of guilt and unworthiness; failure to develop satisfactory relationships; phobias.

Examples of OT techniques: Psychodrama; music therapy; guided fantasy; projective techniques; creative activities.

Criteria for evaluating outcome: The affective state, psychosocial function or symptoms of psychopathology experienced by the individual are observed to have improved and/or the individual reports subjective improvement.

Advantages: Focuses on emotions and relationships; releases unconscious material and makes it accessible; recognizes an irrational basis for behaviour.

Disadvantages: Since the process is highly subjective, it can be hard to define goals or the problem. The process is usually slow; results may not be apparent until months or even years after therapeutic interventions or experiences. The patient may become dependent on the therapist. Traditional Freudian thinking fosters a submissive female stereotype judged by the standards of current western culture (Neo-Freudians have modified accordingly). Psychoanalysis has not been demonstrated to be effective by objective studies (but its practitioners defend this result by saying that objective methods of research are inappropriate and impractical.) For the occupational therapist, the use of dynamic techniques requires expertise. Over-interpretation or misinterpretation by the therapist could be misleading or damaging. Releasing unconscious material without dealing with it appropriately may produce violent emotional reactions and behaviours. Techniques may be stressful for the therapist.

SUGGESTED READING

Books on psychoanalysis are very numerous. The best strategy is to decide which theorist you are interested in and to obtain books by, or about him/her. Psychology books will contain summaries of basic theories.

Balint M 1984 The basic fault. Arrowsmith, Bristol
Bruce M A, Borg B 1987 Frames of reference in psychiatric occupational therapy. Slack, New Jersey (Object relations; frame of reference)
Creek J (ed) 1990 Occupational therapy and mental health: principles, skills and practice. Churchill Livingstone, Edinburgh (ch 13 OT and group psychotherapy)
Finlay L 1988 Occupational therapy practice in psychiatry. Croom Helm, London (ch 2)

Foulkes S H, Anthony E J 1965 Group psychotherapy: the analytical approach. Penguin, Harmondsworth
Mosey A C 1981 Configuration of a profession. Raven Press, New York (ch 14 Analytical frame of reference)
Mosey A C 1986 Psychosocial components of occupational therapy. Raven Press, New York (ch 21 & ch 22 Analytical frame of reference)
Reed K L 1984 Models of practice in occupational therapy. Williams & Wilkins, Baltimore (ch 6 Supermodels; object relations)
Willson M 1984 Occupational therapy in short term psychiatry, 2nd edn. Churchill Livingstone, Edinburgh

THE INTERACTIVE APPROACH

In psychiatric settings, there are two aspects to the interactive approach, which may or may not overlap: firstly, a concern with the individual's skills of interpersonal communication, and secondly, a concern with the ability of an individual to function as a member of a group, and the power of the group to function as a therapeutic entity.

In social skills training, the therapist will assess deficits in verbal and non-verbal communication, personal appearance and cultural appropriateness and will design situations and exercises which will promote the ability of the patient to initiate and sustain appropriate and effective interactions with other individuals, to recognize and express his own needs and to take account of the needs of others. This experience is based on cognitive and experiential methods, not behavioural ones. This approach may also include skills training, particularly social interactive skills, communication skills and skills in assertion. This may begin dyadically with individuals who are unable to cope with being in a group, but such techniques are most often used in a group.

In group therapy, the interactive approach uses theories of group dynamics and may borrow or adapt techniques derived from psychotherapeutic practice. There is a wide spectrum of types of groups, from relatively unstructured, open groups, with a rapid turnover in participants and often arranged around the focus of a social or activity based theme, to closed psychotherapy groups which operate over an extended period with a fixed number of participants, and which may or may not involve task-related activity.

It is typical of this form of group work that the product of group activity, whilst giving the group a focus and a potential sense of achievement, is subordinate to the group process, which provides the insights and learning experiences for group members and gives the therapist opportunities to explore group dynamics. However, whilst there may be a degree of interpretation and analysis of the dynamics of interactions or the results of participation in activities, the main purpose of the group is to provide opportunities for members to participate, in order to explore their personal re-

actions and problems by means of interactions and shared group processes or to improve their abilities to communicate their own needs and to be sensitive to those of others.

Summary of the interactive approach

Metamodel: Although the deterministic effects of unconscious material and drives are acknowledged, this approach tends to be undogmatic. It is holistic in the sense that it is concerned with the individual's perception of reality and reactions to, and communication with others; but analysis may also be carried out. This approach is often a pragmatic — if philosophically unsound — synthesis of ideas and techniques which accepts both metamodels as valid.

Origin of problem: Because of past bad experiences, lack of opportunities, lack of skills, personality disorders, psychiatric disorders or faulty perceptions of reality, the individual is unable to identify or to express his own needs and wishes, to form relationships, to communicate with others or to take account of the needs and wishes of others.

Primary assumptions
- The skills of interacting with other people can only be acquired experientially. Role play, rehearsal and modelling assist skill development.
- Interaction with other people in structured therapeutic groups provides a means of achieving personal growth and insight and developing interactive skills.
- The group process is in itself a dynamic and potent therapeutic medium.
- Personal growth is a painful process which requires a secure and supportive group environment.
- Group work can facilitate communication and cohesion between group members and provides a means of dealing with conflicts.

Terminology: Client; therapist; cotherapist; group leader; facilitator; closed group; open group; group process; group dynamic.

Examples of applications: Interactive techniques are used with a great variety of people, e.g. staff groups, support groups, carer groups, as well as for the treatment of psychiatric conditions. Group work is not normally used with people who are highly disturbed, hyperactive or producing very challenging or disruptive behaviour.

Examples of techniques: Role play; 'gaming'; projective techniques; psychodrama; creative activities; assertion training; anxiety management; stress management; communication skills training; social skills training (cognitive base, not behavioural).

Criteria for evaluating outcome: The individual shows improved awareness of himself and others and improved abilities to express his own needs and meet those of others.

Advantages: When well-led or facilitated, group work can produce good results. Working with people in groups is an effective use of resources.

The group process is experiential and highly relevant to the client; although beneficial results may be slow to appear they tend to be long lasting.

Disadvantages: A group needs to meet several times to be effective. A therapeutic group may need to continue for several months and results may not appear until long after the group is ended. Group management — whichever style of leadership or facilitation is employed — is highly skilled. Group work is stressful for the therapist, who must have access to proper supervision. Although analysis is not usually the main purpose, group processes can produce unexpected and potentially explosive reactions if unconscious material surfaces unexpectedly, and this must be dealt with correctly.

SUGGESTED READING

Bion W R 1961 Experiences in groups. Tavistock Publications, London

Creek J (ed) 1990 Occupational therapy and mental health: principles, skills and practice. Churchill Livingstone, Edinburgh   (ch 14 Drama and OT; ch 15 Social skills training)

Douglas T 1976 Groupwork in practice. Tavistock Publications, London.

Gerard B A, Boniface W J, Howe B H 1980 Interpersonal skills for health professionals. Reston, Virginia

Heap K 1979 Process and action in working with groups. Pergamon Press, Oxford

Hopkins H L, Smith H D (eds) 1988 Willard & Spackman's occupational therapy. Lippincott, Philadelphia   (ch 20, Sections 1 & 2)

Howe M C, Shwartzenburg S L 1986 A functional approach to group work in occupational therapy. Lippincott, Philadelphia

Mosey A C 1986 Psychosocial components of occupational therapy. Raven Press, New York   (ch 12, 13, 14 Groups)

Reed K L 1984 Models of practice in occupational therapy. Williams & Wilkins, Baltimore   (ch 13 Intra and interpersonal performance models)

Remocker A J, Storch E T 1982 Action speaks louder. Churchill Livingstone, Edinburgh

Robertson E 1984 The role of the occupational therapist in a psychotherapeutic setting. British Journal of Occupational Therapy 47 (4): 106–110

Willson M 1984 Occupational therapy in short term psychiatry. Churchill Livingstone, Edinburgh

Yallom I D 1975 Theory and practice of group psychotherapy. Basic Books, New York

Yallom I D 1983 In-patient group psychotherapy. Basic Books, New York

Whittaker D S 1985 Using groups to help people. Routledge & Kegan Paul, London

THE HUMANIST FRAME OF REFERENCE

Humanism is a philosophy rather than a psychological theory, having links with both western existentialism and oriental philosophies concerned with the expansion of consciousness. Humanists consider it essential to take an holistic view of the individual and they prize personal experiences and openness to one's own feelings. There are many natural resonances between humanism and the fundamental philosophy of occupational therapy, as expressed by its American founders.

Influential theorists are Maslow (self-actualization), Frankl (personal meaning), Kelly (personal

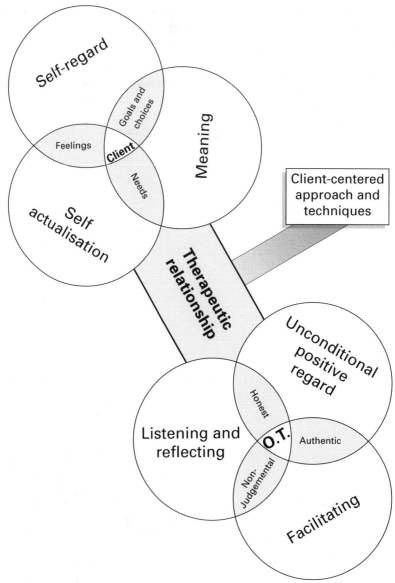

Fig. 2.5 The humanist frame of reference.

constructs) and Rogers (person-centred counselling). Humanists emphasize the essentially positive nature of every individual, who should be valued and will respond accordingly. The individual has the potential to control his life and to choose what he wishes to become. He can only change and progress if he wills to do so; change can only take place if it is an active process which is meaningful to the individual. Positive change can occur throughout life. Living should be a celebratory, joyful experience. Whilst some humanists take an atheistic standpoint, others combine humanism with Christianity or other religious beliefs.

Important concepts in the humanist view of

personal relationships are the need for authenticity — being one's true self — honesty, and non-judgemental regard and respect for others. These theories have become influential in psychotherapy, teaching, social work and OT, linking particularly with some developmental and cognitive theories.

Rogers has been very significant in the move from teacher/therapist centred, directive approaches to student/client centred ones: therapists should act as counsellors or facilitators, providing resources and enabling people to learn and change. Learning is seen as a life long search for individual meaning, fulfilment, growth and self-knowledge. Rogers' ideas are based on personal experience as a teacher and counsellor, backed up by the anecdotal accounts of others. Key features of Rogerian counselling are that it is client centred, using a non-directive style. Interpretation is avoided and the client's ideas, perceptions and beliefs are reflected back, providing encouragement for the individual to search for personal meaning and self-actualization. Humanists believe that it is theoretically possible, by means of counselling, for an individual to achieve a large degree of self-knowledge and control over his own life.

Humanism has been criticized for promoting unrealistic starry-eyed optimism and, whilst the ideals are given lip service by many, they are frequently not put into practice — not least because many of the systems within which health care is delivered make it difficult to allow the amount of time and the degree of freedom of choice for the client which is required. In reality, the opportunity for the individual to control, direct and shape his own life may be minimal and whilst choice may be beneficial, some clients are overwhelmed by being presented with too much of it. The amount of expertise and training required to use humanistic techniques such as client centred counselling is also frequently underestimated: whilst basic counselling skills can be acquired quite readily by most therapists, it should be recognized that clients requiring long term or in-depth counselling should be referred to a suitably qualified counsellor or psychotherapist.

A number of holistic, humanist-style psychotherapies have evolved, frequently combining elements of cognitive or developmental theories with humanism and psychotherapy. These include:

- Gestalt therapy (Perls)
- Rational emotive therapy (Ellis)
- Personal construct (repertory grid) (Kelly; Bannister & Fransella)
- Transactional analysis (Berne)
- Psychosynthesis (Assagioli)
- Person centred counselling (Maslow; Rogers)
- Encounter groups (Rogers)
- Co-counselling (Jackins)
- Theme centred group work (Cohn)

In the context of occupational therapy, humanism has given rise to the *client centred approach*, in which the client is encouraged to direct her own therapy as far as may be possible, to accept personal responsibility and to make decisions. Aims of treatment and activities are selected by the client and must have some personal meaning for her.

Summary of the humanist client centred approach

Metamodel: Strongly holistic.

Origin of problem: The individual is dysfunctional because of damage, developmental disorder, lack of opportunity to acquire skill, lack of the information required to make correct choices, environmental stress, failure to achieve, poor self-actualization, lack of positive regard from others, poor self-esteem, or a combination of such factors.

Primary assumptions
- The personal experience and consciousness of the individual is of paramount importance; since no one else can experience these, no one should attempt to influence another's choices or interpretations of reality.
- The individual must be considered as a whole in the context of his physical and social environment.
- An individual has the right to personal choice (and all other human rights).

- The goal of the individual is to be autonomous, authentic and self-actualizing (functioning as a free, self-directing, honest person whose life brings self-satisfaction and contains personal meaning).
- The individual is capable of controlling events in his life and should direct his own education or therapy as far as possible.
- An individual is innately capable of positive development.

Terminology: Client; facilitator; counsellor; person centred therapy; counselling; self-directed learning, authenticity; self-actualization.

Client/therapist relationship: Central to humanism is the rejection of power being exercised by one person over another. Therapy must be client centred and the therapist must ensure that control is given to the client, even at the expense of very slow decision-taking. The therapist acts as facilitator, providing opportunities and information to enable the client to decide what he wants, and then arranging the resources or intervention to achieve this. Sometimes, a mutual contract is agreed. Where a client is incapable of making his own choices, someone should act as his advocate, putting forward his wishes in so far as they can be ascertained and attempting to put the client's viewpoint as he might have done himself.

Examples of application: The client centred approach can be used with any individual.

Examples of associated OT techniques: Counselling; group work and role play; client centred rehabilitation or education; assertion training; creative therapies; guided fantasy; drama; relaxation; yoga; meditation.

Although the therapist may select techniques which facilitate the client's opportunities for choice and self-expression if the client is temporarily or, by nature of his dysfunction, unable to do so, selection of techniques should normally be negotiated between the client and the therapist, or selected by the client.

Criteria for evaluation of outcome: The client accepts that whatever outcomes he set for himself or negotiated with the therapist have been achieved, or that the need for the therapist's intervention has ended.

Advantages: As a general philosophy of care, it is widely applicable. It is a dynamic, holistic, flexible approach which can deal with psychological, developmental and physical dysfunction, and with deteriorating and terminal conditions. As a method of counselling or teaching, the process is client directed and it is therefore perceived as highly relevant; motivation is positive and results tend to be permanent.

Disadvantages: It can be slow, goals can be 'fuzzy' and it may, if taken too literally, be so non-directive that nothing happens and the process can be 'all talk, no do'. This approach may not be comfortably compatible with the central 'occupations and activities' concerns of occupational therapy, in which case the client would be better referred to a counsellor. The concept of a person being able to control all the choices in his life may be overstated and unrealistic. Interventions can be hard to evaluate so that evidence of success is often anecdotal.

SUGGESTED READING

There is a large amount of literature and you should aim to track down books by the particular theorist in whom you are interested. Because the philosophy of humanism is closely related to that of occupational therapy, some books discussing humanistic theory are listed below, in addition to the OT references.

Abraham B 1988 The dilemmas of helping someone towards independence; an experiential account. British Journal of Occupational Therapy 51: 8 pp 277–279

Eagan G 1986 The skilled helper. Brooks Cole, California

Finlay L 1988 Occupational therapy practice in psychiatry. Croom Helm, London (ch 2)

Kirshenbaum H, Henderson V L (eds) 1990 Carl Rogers dialogues. Constable, London

Kirschenbaum H, Henderson V L (eds) 1990 The Carl Rogers reader. Constable, London

Maslow A H 1968 Towards a psychology of being. Van

Nostrad, New York

Maslow A H 1970 Motivation and personality. Harper & Row, New York

Rogers C 1984 Client centred therapy: its current practice, implications and theory. Houghton Miffin, Boston

Rogers C 1986 On becoming a person. Constable, London

Willson M 1984 Occupational therapy in short term psychiatry. Churchill Livingstone, Edinburgh (ch 4 Humanistic psychology)

Willson M 1987 Occupational therapy in long term psychiatry. Churchill Livingstone, Edinburgh (ch 2 Humanistic influence)

How directive are you?

By the end of this chapter, it will have become apparent that one of the central issues in the application of frames of reference is the degree to which the therapist or the patient/client has control of the therapeutic situation.

The spectrum is very wide — all the way from a highly structured behavioural modification programme in which every aspect is controlled by the therapist to the completely client centred approach in which the client selects his own therapy and takes a large amount of personal responsibility for it.

Many therapists would strongly deny being directive — very probably, this includes you. But it is all too easy to remove opportunities for control from the patient. This is particularly so when you are working within the constraints of some kind of system which can insidiously begin to dominate the decision taking process.

Consider this example

Mrs Brown has had a hip replacement operation, and has been referred to OT on the ward round following her operation. She is doing well. The therapist visits Mrs Brown on the ward and finds her in the day room in conversation with another patient. The action continues as follows:

THERAPIST: Good morning Mrs Brown, can I interrupt a moment? My name is Miss Green, I'm the occupational therapist. I won't keep you long. (*Brief pause whilst she establishes eye contact with Mrs Brown, who stops talking and pays attention; so does other patient.*)

THERAPIST: How are you feeling after your operation?

MRS B: Rather sore, and I'm due to have my stitches out. But I did walk here from my bed without the nurse helping me.

THERAPIST: Fine. Mr Sawbone has asked me to see you; he says you are doing well and he hopes you can go home in a few days. I'd like you to come down to the occupational therapy department this afternoon so that I can tell you how best to manage with your new hip.

MRS B: Will that be after visiting time?

THERAPIST: Oh yes, you should be back in time. Oh, and can you bring some everyday clothes down with you?

MRS B: Yes, alright.

THERAPIST: Fine, I'll see you later then. (*Smiles at Mrs B and friend and leaves.*)

Now try this exercise

Either write down, or discuss in pairs or in a small group:

1 How would you change the script?
2 How is control removed from Mrs Brown and how might it be given to her?
3 Taking examples from your current work, can you identify times when you, or someone you have watched, has taken control away from a patient? Was this intentional or not? How could it have been avoided?
4 Are there any systems or policies operating in your area which contribute to the removal of patient control and choice? Are there any which deliberately seek to extend the opportunities for these?
5 How practical is it, in your field of work/clinical placement, to be humanistic in your approach? What are the constraints?

3

Problem based models

In using these models, the therapist has made some preliminary assumptions about the nature of the problem which has lead to the referral of the patient. It is firstly assumed that the patient is dysfunctional, i.e. unable to meet the requirements of his life adaptively and effectively. Secondly, it is assumed that there is a particular cause for this dysfunction, and it is this cause which leads to the selection of the relevant model.

A dysfunction is a temporary or chronic inability to engage in the roles, relationships and occupations expected of a person of comparable age, sex and culture. Note that this is not the same as a *disability*; the latter tends to imply a loss of physical ability, but one may be dysfunctional without having any kind of physical impairment or injury, and equally one may be disabled (e.g. a paraplegic or an amputee), but capable of leading a very functional and adaptive life. (Dysfunction, disability, handicap and impairment is another set of words with multiple definitions; see Glossary.)

In the *rehabilitation model*, it is assumed that the patient was previously able, but that function has been lost as a result of illness or injury. ('Was able — now can't do'.)

In the *development model*, it is assumed that the patient is not functional because he has not yet reached the developmental level which would enable him to become so. ('Is not yet able — can't yet do'.)

In the *education model*, the origin of the problem is viewed as lack of skill, knowledge, appropriate attitude or experience, although the basic ability to become functional is present. ('Would be able — doesn't know how to'.)

All three models are fundamentally optimistic in outlook. It is implicit that given the right treatment/training/education, the patient's level of function will improve. These models are integrative, in that they coordinate the use of compatible treatment approaches and techniques. The models are also complementary to each other; in practice, it is possible to change the emphasis from one model to another during different parts of the treatment process.

In the interests of comparison and consistency, similar headings have been used to summarize these models as were used to summarize approaches, but it should be remembered that, as previously suggested, models operate at a different level of organization to approaches.

THE REHABILITATION MODEL

Rehabilitation has been defined by the World Health Organization as, 'the combined and coordinated use of medical, social, educational and vocational measures for training or retraining the individual to the highest possible level of functional ability' (WHO 1974).

The WHO further distinguishes between medical, social and vocational rehabilitation, as follows:

Medical rehabilitation: The process of medical care aiming at developing the functional and psychological abilities of the individual and, if necessary, his compensatory mechanisms, so as to enable him to attain self-dependence and lead an active life.

Social rehabilitation: That part of the rehabilitation process aimed at the integration or reintegration of a disabled person into society by helping him to adjust to the demands of family, community and occupation while reducing any economic or social burdens that may impede the total rehabilitation process.

Vocational rehabilitation: The provision of those vocational services, e.g. vocational guidance, vocational training and selective placement, designed to enable a disabled person to secure and retain suitable employment.

(WHO 1974)

In British practice, the rehabilitation model is still one of the most widely used and the majority of British OT textbooks on physical disabilities written before 1980 have, in the main, been based upon it (Jones 1964; McDonald 1964; Jones & Jay 1977).

The aims of rehabilitation are well defined:

- To enable the individual to achieve independence in the areas of work and self-care.
- To restore the individual's functional ability to the previously attained level, or as close to this as possible.
- To maximize and maintain the potential of retained, undamaged, abilities.
- To compensate for residual disability by means of aids, appliances, orthoses or environmental adaptations.

The process of rehabilitation requires a detailed knowledge of the patient's medical, social and environmental circumstances. Aims of treatment must be geared closely to the needs of the individual. Methods include use of techniques drawn from the biomechanical, neurodevelopmental, cognitive, behavioural, interactive and, more recently, client centred approaches.

As implied by the WHO definition, rehabilitation is normally viewed as an interdisciplinary process, in which members of a team bring together skills appropriate to the needs of the patient and work in close cooperation to achieve jointly agreed rehabilitative goals.

The strongest focuses of physical rehabilitation have traditionally been on the restoration of sensori-motor function, independence in activities of daily living (ADL), work skills and social skills. Rehabilitation is also used as a model in psychiatry, particularly in the preparation of people who have become institutionalized and de-skilled through very long stays in hospital or through the effects of severe psychotic illness.

Summary of the rehabilitation model

Metamodel: The model is nominally holistic, and the importance of taking a broadly based view of the patient and her needs, and of considering

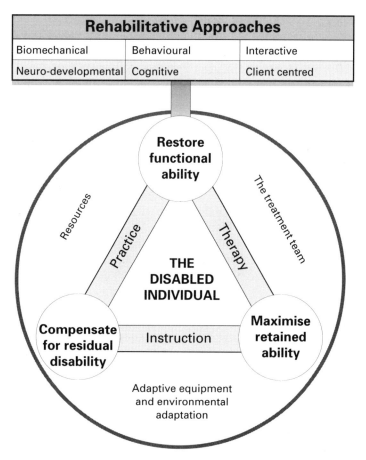

Fig. 3.1 The rehabilitation model.

ability as well as disability, is often stressed in the literature. It has to be admitted, however, that in practice, probably because of its long association with the medical model and because of the constraints on available treatment time, the model can become reductionist, homing in on the lost function and excluding the wider issues. This is particularly so in fast flow physical rehabilitation when using a biomechanical approach.

Origin of the problem: The patient has lost a previous ability (or abilities) due to illness or trauma.

Primary assumptions

- Therapy should promote personal independence and should restore function to normal or near normal.

- Restoration of function can be achieved by graded practice of the damaged ability.
- Retraining should be carried out under realistic conditions with a view to the eventual resettlement location, social situation or work of the patient.
- Where residual disability persists, this may be compensated for by teaching the patient new skills or through the provision of aids, appliances, environmental adaptations or assistance from someone else.

Terminology: Therapist; patient (client when in the community); ability/disability; handicap; dependence/independence; therapy; treatment; rehabilitation.

Patient/therapist relationship: The patient must actively cooperate and be involved in her rehabilitation: the success of rehabilitation is dependent on the skill with which the therapist can build a therapeutic relationship and motivate the patient to participate. Although this relationship is a partnership, traditionally the therapist tends to be the controlling partner, prescribing, advising and providing resources (another legacy of the medical model). However, a humanistic attitude is becoming more common, encouraging the client/patient to direct the rehabilitation process and to select and prioritize personal goals.

Application: The rehabilitation model can be used to treat physical illness or injury, or pyschiatric illness.

Examples of associated approaches: Biomechanical; neurodevelopmental; cognitive; behavioural; interactive; client centred.

Examples of associated techniques: One of the strengths of the model is that it is compatible with many techniques: the danger is that too many techniques may be combined at one time, thus leading to therapeutic inconsistency. For example, it would not be effective to combine biomechanical and neurodevelopmental techniques in physical rehabilitation. (If you are still not sure why, review the section on these approaches.) Because the rehabilitation model evolved early in the history of professional practice, it is also closely associated with the core skills of the profession — particularly assessment, adaptation of occupations, activities and tasks, and environmental adaptation.

Examples of specific techniques

Physical rehabilitation
Assessment and retraining of activities of daily living
Provision of aids and home adaptations
Graded physical/cognitive/perceptual rehabilitation programmes (using biomechanical, cognitive or neurodevelopmental approaches)
Specific prescription of remedial activities
Work retraining and resettlement
Prescription and provision of orthoses
Prosthetic training

Psychiatric rehabilitation
Assessment of social and self-care skills
Social skills training
Behavioural modification
Specific activities to redevelop cognitive, social, self-care or creative skills
Industrial therapy, work retraining and resettlement
Preparation for community living (group homes and hostels)

Criteria for evaluation of outcome: The lost function has been demonstrated to be restored to a normal (or acceptable) level and/or a satisfactory method of compensating for residual disability has been found. The patient has been resettled in a normal or adapted domestic and/or work environment.

Advantages: A positive approach, aiming to improve necessary abilities, maximize existing function and compensate for deficits. Highly practical and good at problem solving. A valuable, well understood, team approach.

Disadvantages: Because of its innately optimistic assumption of improvement, this model copes less well with deteriorating, chronic or terminal conditions. It is also inapplicable in the context of learning disorders, since here it is a matter of 'habilitation', and the education or development models are more appropriate. There may be a tendency to focus on the lost abilities, rather than on those which still exist. If application is allowed to become reductionist, only the obvious problems may be tackled, perhaps dealing with effects rather than causes or failing to take account of psychological problems in a physical setting: skills tend to be dealt with rather than roles or relationships. If overly prescriptive, the patient may be pressed to comply with action which is not her first choice. However, the fact that this model has stood the test of time better than most indicates that it has relatively few disadvantages.

SUGGESTED READING

Bumphrey E (ed) 1987 Occupational therapy in the community. Woodhead & Faulkener, Cambridge
Creek J (ed) 1990 Occupational therapy and mental health: principles, skills and practice. Churchill Livingstone, Edinburgh ch 19 Long stay psychiatry; ch 20 Rehabilitation)
Goodwill C J, Chamberlain M A (eds) 1988 Rehabilitation of the physically disabled adult. Croom Helm, London
Hume C, Pullen M 1986 Rehabilitation in psychiatry. Churchill Livingstone, Edinburgh
Jones M, Jay P (eds) 1977 An approach to occupational therapy, 3rd edn. Butterworths, Sevenoaks
Turner A (ed) 1987 The practice of occupational therapy, 2nd edn. Churchill Livingstone, Edinburgh
Turner A (ed) 1991 The principles, skills and practice of occupational therapy. Churchill Livingstone, Edinburgh
Watts F, Bennett D (eds) 1981 Principles of psychiatric rehabilitation. Wiley, Chichester.
Willson M 1984 Occupational therapy in long term psychiatry. Churchill Livingstone, Edinburgh
Wing J K, Morris B (eds) 1981 Handbook of psychiatric rehabilitation. Oxford University Press, Oxford

THE DEVELOPMENT MODEL

The development model describes the sequence in which learning or development takes place, and usually explains development as an hierarchical process in which one stage has to be completed before progressing to the next.

The first eighteen or so years of human life follow a genetically programmed developmental sequence leading to maturation. Developmental stages are innate, but the extent to which they are achieved depends on environmental influences and opportunities. The 'nature v. nurture' debate remains unresolved: in the past decade, environmental influences have been emphasized, but recent studies comparing identical twins reared in differing environments suggests that genetic factors may be more important than previously thought. Subsequent adult development is a matter of learning opportunities and experiences, and the individual's ability to adapt. Adaptive change over the course of time is called *ontogenesis*. The ability to adapt has positive survival value.

Educationally, developmental theory is of use in looking at the way children learn and acquire skills (motor, perceptual, cognitive, social). The work of Piaget is important in this regard. In the context of adult learning, theories deal more with the sequence in which cognitive abilities and concepts are developed and refined (e.g. Perry; Bruner)

Physiologically, developmental theories are concerned with the maturation of the central nervous system and the sequence of acquisition of neuro-muscular control, proprioceptive discrimination and perceptual skills.

Incomplete, retarded, or dysfunctional development is very significant to the therapist. In therapy, the goal is frequently that of retracing the pattern of development in order to advance the level of an individual's skills (see neuro-developmental approach).

Summary of the development model

Metamodel: Apart from the deterministic aspects of genetic inheritance, the model is holistic, viewing the individual as a complex organism in whom all parts are interrelated, and on whom the environment also has an influence.

Origin of problem: Dysfunction is due to incomplete, retarded or maladaptive development, or to the effects of stress or trauma which may have caused the individual to regress to a more primitive developmental level.

Primary assumptions
- All individuals have developmental potential.
- The individual develops (physically, intellectually, emotionally, socially) in a defined sequence related to age.
- Stages in the developmental sequence can not be missed or jumped if the individual is to function within the norms for his age.
- The individual cannot function at a higher level than his stage of development. (But some authorites accept that it is possible to

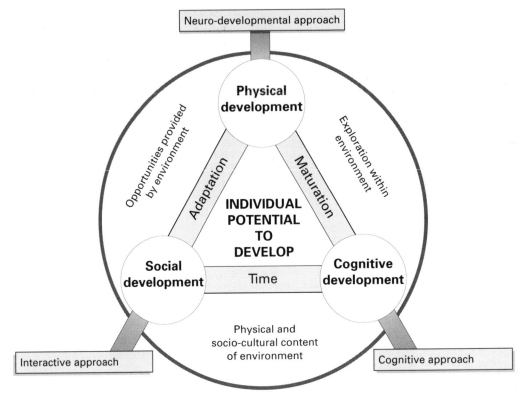

Fig. 3.2 The development model.

develop unevenly, and to be mature in some respects but not in others.)

- Environment, experience and opportunity limits, or maximizes, the extent to which developmental potential can be fulfilled.

Terminology: Therapist; patient/client; adaptation/maladaptation; function/dysfunction; development sequence/levels; therapy; intervention.

Patient/therapist relationship: This is affected by the age and degree of dysfunction of the patient, and there is a wide continuum, from the therapist being strongly controlling and directive, to a partnership between therapist and patient. Because the therapist has to work within a developmental framework which implies setting quite precise objectives for therapy, some degree of prescriptive control is inevitable.

Examples of applications: Psychiatric disorders; neurological disorders; sensori-motor disorders; learning difficulties; paediatric disorders.

Examples of associated approaches: Neuro-developmental; cognitive (cognitive/behavioural); interactive.

Examples of techniques

Physical dysfunction
Diagnostic assessment of physical and perceptual developmental levels; Sensory integration (Ayres)
Neurodevelopmental techniques (Bobath; Rood; PNF; conductive education); Environmental adaptation to promote development

Learning difficulties (mental handicap)
Neurodevelopmental techniques
Portage
Sensory integration
Sensory stimulation (special environments)
Developmentally based special education

Psychiatric disorders
Diagnostic assessment of developmental levels (Mosey; Allen)
Sensory integration (King)

Development of adaptive skills (Mosey)

Activities to promote cognitive/perceptual development

Criteria for evaluation of outcome: The individual has achieved the normal developmental level for his/her age/sex or has shown progression from one level to a more advanced one.

Advantages: The development model is based on well researched physiological and psychological theories, It is optimistically progressive, and can benefit people with low abilities and severe learning deficits, as well as those who have regressed to a lower developmental level as a result of illness, trauma or stress.

Disadvantages: Working developmentally can be slow and usually requires intensive therapy. The therapist must be confident and thoroughly competent when working neurodevelopmentally, where effective application requires expert use of technique. This takes practice, experience and a sound comprehension of the basic theory. Progress can be retarded or lost unless all members of the team use the same techniques consistently. This model is not appropriate for deteriorating or terminal conditions (although some of the associated techniques may be).

SUGGESTED READING

Bruce M A, Borg B 1987 Frames of reference in psychiatric occupational therapy. Slack, New Jersey (Developmental frame of reference)
Hopkins H L, Smith H D (eds) 1988 Willard & Spackman's occupational therapy, 7th edn. Lippincott, Philadelphia (ch 4; ch 8, sections 1, 2, 3)
Mosey A C 1981 Occupational therapy: configuration of a profession. Raven Press, New York (ch 14 Developmental frame of reference)
Mosey A C 1986 Psychosocial components of occupational therapy. Raven Press, New York (ch 23 Developmental frame of reference; ch 24 Recapitulation of ontogensis)

Trombley C A 1983 Occupational therapy for physical dysfunction, 2nd edn. Williams & Wilkins, Baltimore (ch 6 Neurodevelopmental techniques)
Pedretti L (ed) 1985 Occupational therapy: practice skills for physical dysfunction, 2nd edn. Mosby, St Louis (ch 13, 14, 15, 16, 17 Neurodevelopmental techniques)
Reed K L 1984 Models of practice in occupational therapy. Williams & Wilkins, Baltimore (Developmental, neurodevelopmental and neuroperceptual models)
Willson M 1987 Occupational therapy in long-term psychiatry. Churchill Livingstone, Edinburgh (ch 4 Developmental approaches)

THE EDUCATION MODEL

Some occupational therapists reject the education model on the basis that they are *therapists*, not teachers. While that is true, it would be misleading to say that therapists do not teach: many spend much of their time doing so, but often in an informal, unstructured manner which may be so subliminal that both therapist and client fail to recognize the process.

In other cases, education is more formal and readily identified. Education of colleagues and other professionals, health education for the general public and student education and supervision, are all important and integral parts of the therapist's role.

Perhaps some of the misunderstandings arise from the fact that the therapist deals mainly with *adult* learners (paediatrics excepted). This has been called *andragogy* (Knowles) as distinct from pedagogy.

Moreover, the therapist deals frequently with adults who have special learning needs. There has been considerable research into adult learning styles and appropriate methods of teaching adults, the more recent of which tends to emphasize the importance of moving towards student centred and experiential styles of learning, rather than teacher centred instruction. However, except in the case of special needs or remedial teaching, where the boundaries between therapist and

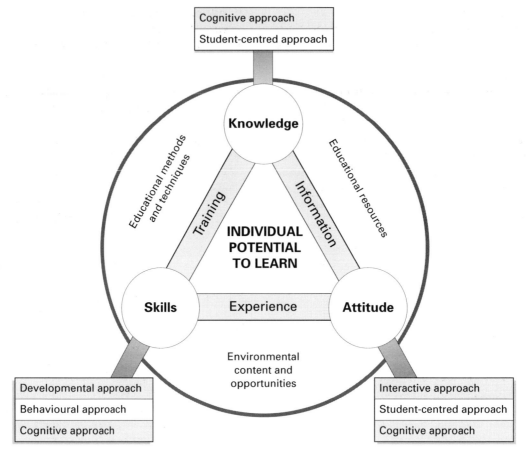

Fig. 3.3 The education model.

teacher truly blur, the therapist has a different basis for the use of educational techniques and differing concerns from those of the teacher.

Theories of learning and teaching techniques are derived from the frames of reference previously discussed:

- *Physiological*: researching into the neurophysiology of learning.
- *Behavioural*: breaking down complex behaviour into skills and subskills and viewing learning as a product of environmental reward and reinforcement.
- *Cognitive*: viewing learning as dependent on cognitive processes (remembering, processing, storing, retrieving) which then direct behaviour.

- *Developmental*: seeing learning as a sequential process, building on experience.
- *Humanistic*: emphasizing that one cannot teach another person, only facilitate his experiential self-directed learning.

One of the few things on which the opposing theorists agree is that learning is fundamental to human behaviour. The debate over how one should define learning or behaviour, how an individual learns, what is learnt or which is the best method of ensuring that learning takes place, has filled many educational textbooks.

A definition of learning is 'the relatively permanent changes in potential for performance that result from past interactions with the environment' (Lovell). Learning is distinguished from changes due to basic physical maturation, although the individual has to learn in order to make best use of the potentials which come with each stage of maturation.

What is learnt is commonly divided into knowledge, skills and attitudes. Therapists often need to increase a person's knowledge, improve his skills or change his attitudes. Educational theorists discuss the differences between these types of learning, and suggest differing ways of teaching each type. There are many similarities between the process of education — requiring aims, objectives and methods of achieving these — and the process of therapy.

Other educational researchers have explored the ways in which people learn, both as children and adults, dealing with learning styles and strategies and with the physiological basis for learning.

In view of the amount of time therapists spend attempting to produce 'relatively permanent changes in potential for performance', it is surprising to find that few OT textbooks devote much, if any, space on educational theory as such. One has to scan the indexes and read selectively. There is, on the other hand, an overwhelming amount of educational literature.

Summary of the education model

Metamodel: The education model can be either holistic or reductionist, depending on the approach being used.

Origin of problem: The client/patient/learner has failed to learn because of a cognitive deficit, learning difficulty or lack of opportunity, experience or instruction. Inadequate, incomplete or incorrect learning results in a lack of knowledge or lack of skill, or an inappropriate attitude — leading to deficits in performance or behaviour.

Primary assumptions
- Most human behaviour is learnt (but there are various theoretical explanations of the way in which this occurs).

- Effective learning results in a long-lasting change in behaviour.
- It is possible to improve knowledge or skills or to develop attitudes by providing appropriate teaching, practice or experience.
- Given time and the right techniques, all but the most severely brain damaged individuals are capable of some learning.

Terminology: Client/patient/student/learner/trainee; therapist/trainer/teacher/instructor; teaching/training/instructing/demonstrating/educating; learning objectives; skills; competencies.

Learner/therapist relationship: Reductionist approaches — the therapist controls and directs; the student learns, actively or passively.
Holistic approaches — student centred. The therapist facilitates or teaches; the student learns actively and may direct the whole process.

Examples of educational approaches: Physiological; behavioural; cognitive; developmental; student centred.

Examples of techniques
Physiological, e.g. training motor skills and perceptual-motor skills; biofeedback.
Behavioural, e.g. behavioural modification; errorless learning; chaining and backward chaining; habit training; social skills training.
Cognitive, e.g. memory and perceptual training; assertion training; stress management.
Developmental, e.g. conductive education; portage.
Humanist, e.g. student centred learning; experiential learning.

Criteria for evaluating outcome: Learning objectives have been met: there is observed to be a permanent change in the individual's knowledge, skill or attitude as a result of new learning.

Advantages/disadvantages: Methods and contexts are so varied that a brief discussion of advantages and disadvantages is impossible. Possibly the main disadvantage is that any learning process takes time and learners experiencing difficulties require a large amount of individual attention if learning is to be effective.

SUGGESTED READING

These publications are particularly helpful to a therapist, and deal with adult learning. If you wish to pursue this topic further, you will find many more references in the books themselves.

Bandura A 1977 Social learning theory, Prentice Hall, New Jersey

Bigge M 1987 Learning theories for teachers, 4th edn. Harper & Row, New York

Gagné R M 1977 The conditions of learning and theory of instruction, 3rd edn. Holt Saunders, Eastbourne (Cognitive/behavioural approach)

Knowles M 1978 The adult learner: a neglected species. Gulf, Houston

Lovell R B 1987 Adult learning. Croom Helm, London (Basic review of theories)

Mocellin G 1988 A perspective on the principles and practice of occupational therapy. British Journal of Occupational Therapy 51:1 pp 4–7

Rogers C 1983 Freedom to learn for the 80s. Charles E Merrill, Columbus, Ohio

Watts N T 1990 Handbook of clinical teaching. Churchill Livingstone, Edinburgh (Subtitled 'Exercises and guidelines for health professionals who teach patients, train staff or supervise students')

The three models just discussed are widely used across the whole spectrum of OT practice. Probably you use one or more yourself or have seen them in use. With a colleague, or in a small group, discuss the following questions using your own experience to provide illustrations.

1 Why is it useful to distinguish between the three suggested causes of dysfunction?

2 From your current case load, select a patient who would fit one of the causational assumptions. Are you treating him/her within the model as I have described it? How did you decide which techniques to use? Are you 'mixing and matching', moving in and out of more than one model in the course of therapy? Would a more structured application of a model improve the effectiveness of your therapy?

3 How far should therapists act as trainers or educators? Do therapists make good use of educators and educational theory?

THE PROBLEM SOLVING MODEL

Problem solving as a process is widely used by occupational therapists. It is therefore surprising to find that very little has been written about it in the professional literature. Perhaps it appears to be too much like stating the obvious, or perhaps it is not conceptualized as a model. Problem solving as a model of practice differs from other models in two important respects. Whereas with other models one has already 'put on the coloured spectacles' or 'selected the tool' (i.e. decided on the nature of the problem and selected an appropriate approach) *before* beginning to assess or treat the patient, with problem solving, one postpones the choice of 'tool' until *after* the assessment of the patient.

Secondly, the problem solving model is a description of a process, rather than a set of theories. The problem solving process is a conscious attempt to avoid the assumptions and blinkered thinking which may be inherent in other models, and to view the patient holistically and objectively before deciding on the nature of the problem and how (or if) to treat it.

Because the model is related to the problem and not to a particular theory, an eclectic selection and synthesis of relevant treatment techniques or approaches can be made, crossing the boundaries of the metamodels (providing that techniques do not clash).

One of the features of the problem solving model is that it may highlight the fact that the 'problem' does not lie with the patient, but with her physical or social environment. It is also possible to identify that, although a problem may exist, intervention is unnecessary, ineffective or not beneficial. Whilst problem solving is frequently used informally, there is a more structured and deliberate form of the process which will be described below.

The problem solving process

Data collection

The key to problem solution is gathering sufficient information about the situation. This may occupy much of the time spent on the problem: once it is possible to identify accurately what the problem is, a solution is frequently obvious. Attempting to solve a problem which is inadequately understood, or where too many assumptions have been made, is seldom successful.

Having too much data, however, is often a bigger difficulty than having too little — the ability to select the relevant from the irrelevant comes with experience. Expert judgement and knowledge may be required. The creation of 'expert systems' — computer data bases and diagnostic programmes aimed at helping with clinical problem solving — is a recent development to assist doctors and other professionals. So far, there have been few attempts to create expert systems for use by occupational therapists (Arnold & Penn 1990). Information processing is now an important separate branch of knowledge, both in computers and in cognitive psychology.

Problem identification

This involves providing answers to questions such as: What is the problem? Are there more than one? If so, which is the most significant? Which should be tackled first? The apparent or obvious problem may not turn out to be the real cause of the difficulty; action may turn out to be inadvisable or impossible.

The logical sequence in which problems are tackled is also important — effort is wasted by dealing with subsidiary issues which would be resolved by solution of the root cause.

Identification of the desired outcome

Identification of the problem — the 'undesired state' — must bring with it a clear specification of the 'desired state.' This is not the same as a solution, which is the method whereby that state may be achieved, and which may be far more difficult to identify. The desired outcome may be clear, but the route to it very hard to find. Often, there is only one desired outcome, but sometimes there may be alternatives, which can be evaluated for comparative benefits, put in priority order, discarded, or kept in reserve as a viable alternative if the first choice proves unattainable.

Solution development, evaluation and selection

The human brain is uniquely geared to be effective at problem solving. At a low level, it can do this so rapidly that it appears intuitive, although it is actually based on fast processing of previous knowledge and experience, together with insightful connective 'jumps' between pieces of information.

When the problem is complex, the mind generates a series of 'what if' hypotheses and previously learnt 'rules' which seem applicable, and tests these against the desired state. At this stage, production of many possible strategies is more effective than becoming 'hooked' on one or two. Good problem solvers are very flexible, have well developed lateral (divergent) thinking, and use strategies such as 'brain-storming' to produce a multitude of creative and novel solutions.

Evaluation and selection of solutions is another key stage in the process: effectiveness may not be the only criterion. For example, one may need to consider time, resources, effort, cost, practicality, acceptability to the client, and so on. (In management terms this may be referred to as 'cost-benefit analysis'.)

Development of an action plan

The action plan specifies the stages by which the solution will be implemented, and the desired state achieved. It should also make clear who is responsible for doing what. Although the plan should not become too rigid, clarity in specifying the goal, timescale, and method of testing success or failure is helpful.

Implementation. The plan is put into action and the process and results are recorded.

Assessment of results

The effectiveness of the action is measured against progress towards the previously agreed outcome. Once that is achieved, intervention ceases or moves to another problem. Compromises may be necessary. Action may uncover previously unsuspected problems which need to be dealt with. Action which is ineffective must be changed. Was the solution wrong? Was the problem incorrectly defined in the first place? Is the problem insoluble or the gain not worth prolonged effort? Answers to these questions usually require a return circuit round the problem solving process, gathering more information and redefining the problem. Clearly, this process has much in common with the basic treatment process used by therapists and others, but it is more structured and formalized.

Problem based recording systems

Problem solving as a formal model is often associated with problem based systems of recording, particularly problem oriented medical records (POMR) (Weed 1968, 1969) and the SOAP system (Kings Fund Centre 1988) (see below).

Problem oriented medical records

Using this system, the problems experienced by the patient are identified and listed. They may be categorized under headings according to a standardized system, and may be allocated numbers. Once listed, problems are prioritized and may be divided into short term and long term goals. A treatment plan is designed and implemented for selected goals.

It is useful to separate the *treatment plan*, which will involve the patient's direct participation, from the *action plan*, which is what the therapist (or others) will do. All references to the treatment and subsequent progress in resolving the problem refer to it by number. When the problem is resolved, it is removed from the list and a subsequent problem may be tackled (Kings Fund Centre 1988).

Putting this recording system into practice requires some effort and discipline, but once set up

it does aid teamwork and concentrates efforts on practical issues, identifying action to be taken, the most appropriate person to take it, and facilitating review of progress.

SOAP is a method of problem identification and solution. SOAP stands for:

> Subjective
> Objective
> Analysis (or Assessment)
> Planning

First, the patient's subjective view of her situation is obtained and recorded, together with the subjective views of any other people involved. Following this the therapist will identify some likely problem areas and will investigate these objectively, by formal observation and assessments.

The results of these procedures will then be analysed in order to decide what the problem(s) might be. At this stage, it may become clear that the patient's subjective view differs from the objective assessment of the therapist, or from the subjective views of significant others, and this mismatch may, in fact, constitute the problem. Once a problem list has been composed, it is possible to decide on action.

The planning stage involves selecting priorities, goal setting, generating possible solutions and selecting the preferred one, and putting the plan into action. Although SOAP does not contain another stage, it is implicit that the success of the plan is monitored and reviewed and action modified accordingly.

When using this system, all actions by the therapist are recorded with the key letters S–O–A–P. For example, an interview with the patient would be recorded under S; an observation of the occurrence of a particular difficulty would be under O, together with the number of the problem observed; a case conference might be A or P; the treatment plan would be P.

Using this system does take practice and requires a certain mental discipline, but once proficiency is attained it can greatly speed up and simplify the process of keeping treatment records, as well as making goal setting and planning more precise. It also offers the advantage of a measur-

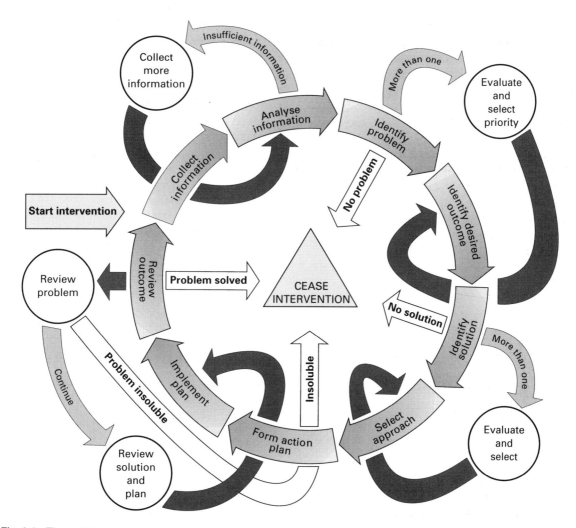

Fig. 3.4 The problem solving model.

able outcome which is of considerable value in implementing quality assurance audits, and producing evidence of the results of therapy.

There can be difficulties in fitting actions or occurrences into the SOAP format, however. Some forms of problem based systems include a 'strengths and needs' assessment of the individual — individual programme planning is an example — so that strengths can be built on as part of the problem solving process. This also avoids the risk of a rather negative 'problem list' which may result in the patient being viewed as 'a problem'.

POMR and SOAP may be linked to a *key worker* system, where an individual is given the responsibility of managing a case and coordinating effective therapy.

Summary of the problem solving model

Metamodel: Pragmatic: it depends on the solution required by the problem.

Origin of the problem: No initial assumptions are made. The problem has first to be defined. This may lead to an explanation, or to one or more solutions for evaluation, and will suggest priorities. The nature of the problem is the key to subsequent action and choice of techniques or approaches.

Primary assumptions

- Adequate data collection is essential for correct analysis of the problem.
- In any problem situation, there may be several applicable solutions — one should keep an open mind.
- Problems should be tackled in an order of priority (but the order may be decided by the patient, or therapist, or pragmatically).
- The apparent problem may not be the real one: the apparent solution may not be the best one.
- Interventions should be goal directed.
- Progress should be monitored and action changed or the problem reassessed if results are ineffective.

Terminology: Patient; client; therapist; problem solving process; goal planning; POMR; SOAP.

Patient/therapist relationship: Depends on the style of the therapist: ranges from directive to client centred. Frequently, the process is negotiated: the therapist assists the client to describe the problem and propose and evaluate solutions. The subsequent role of the patient depends on the selected treatment approach.

Examples of applications: Suitable for all types of patients/clients, particularly where complex situations/conditions are involved. The model is least suited to very straightforward cases, where both problem and solution are instantly obvious.

Treatment techniques/approaches: Anything relevant to the problem, providing mutually incompatible techniques are not used simultaneously.

Problem solving techniques: Problem identification and prioritizing methods used by therapists include: algorithms, flow charts, cognitive mapping, ranking and weighting methods, brainstorming. Crisis intervention in psychiatric emergency may be viewed as a form of team problem-solving to intervene where the client is overwhelmed by major life changes or adverse circumstances.

Problem solving techniques used with patients include scripting, rehearsal, role play, modelling, problem based training, cognitive training.

Criteria for evaluation of outcome: The previously identified 'desired state' has been achieved and the identified problem is resolved.

Advantages: Highly pragmatic, flexible and avoids blinkered thinking. Suitable for all types of patients and can manage deteriorating or complex situations effectively. Promotes teamwork and provides measurable outcomes. Structured recording systems aid communication and evaluation.

Disadvantages: The patient may become viewed as the 'problem'; there may be too much focus on negatives such that strengths and assets may be ignored. Over-eclectic therapy may lack coherence. The whole system relies on very accurate assessment and identification of the problem; incorrect evaluation, wrong priorities or poor solutions render intervention inappropriate or ineffective.

··

Are you a problem solver?

Since problem solving is the basis of most therapeutic processes, I suspect (but have no objective evidence to support this statement) that many OTs use an unstructured form of problem solving, and may, in fact, be using this model when they believe themselves to be using another.

If you are already practising, ask yourself this key question:

'When do I take the decision about how I expect to treat (intervene on behalf of) the patient?'

I suggest that if you view the patient first, undertake subjective and objective collection of information, and *then* make your decision about whether to treat the patient, what needs to be done and how best to do it, you are using problem solving. In that case, a more structured form of the model might enable you to do this more effectively.

If, on the other hand, you meet your patient for her first session with a clear idea of the general direction of your intervention and of the methods you intend to use — for example, you know that you will undertake an ADL assessment and prescribe adaptive equipment, that you will involve your patient in a programme of expressive therapeutic group activities or that you will teach your patient a skill — then you are working within the framework of some other model.

SUGGESTED READING

Gerard B A, Boniface W J, Howe B H 1980 Interpersonal skills for health professionals. Reston, Virginia (section 7 Problem solving)

Hopkins H L, Smith H D (eds) 1988 Willard & Spackman's occupational therapy, 7th edn. Lippincott, Philadelphia (ch 6 Problem solving)

Juniper D F 1989 Successful problem solving. Foulsham, London

Lovell R B 1987 Adult learning. Croom Helm, London (ch 4 Learning cognitive strategies: problem solving)

4

Occupational therapy models

A formal comparative study of the contents of the American and British Journals of Occupational Therapy over the past two decades would undoubtedly be revealing, but as far as I am aware no one has undertaken such a mammoth task. An occasional quick and highly unscientific comparison of contents pages has, however, always left me with the impression that there is a noticeable difference in emphasis and style between practitioners on each side of the Atlantic.

British therapists, when they write about their practice (which is not nearly often enough), tend towards the pragmatic, technical and experiential — the 'whats' and 'hows' of therapy. American therapists on the other hand frequently produce detailed and objective critiques and studies of methods, but also discuss theory and philosophy — the 'whys' of therapy, in a way which their British counterparts, until very recently, have not attempted.

This is not the place to speculate on the educational or cultural differences which account for the differences, but it is not surprising that the most thorough and complex conceptualizations of the profession have originated in the United States where, after all, the profession was founded.

The three models selected for description in this study guide are all based on views of the central importance of occupations in the life of the individual, and their consequent value as therapy.

They share a humanistic, developmental framework and a concern with the skills which people need in order to engage in occupations. Each author seeks to provide an integrated model to direct therapy, a guide to the application of techniques and a means of distinguishing the unique contribution of OT from that of other professions.

The model of human occupation was first published in the *American Journal of Occupational Therapy* by Gary Kielhofner in collaboration with others (Kielhofner & Burke 1980; Kielhofner 1980a & 1980b; Kielhofner & Igi 1980). The ideas have been developed in Kielhofner's book on the model (Kielhofner 1985) and he has continued to refine them: in fact, in some respects, his ideas have changed — a useful reminder that all models are subject to evolution. Kielhofner himself proposed his model as a basis for discussion and development, rather than as a complete and final explanation of OT practice.

The model views a person as an open system interacting with the environment and continually modifying it and being modified by it. The system is arranged as a hierarchy, composed of subsystems: volition (will); habituation (roles, rules); performance (skill). It focuses on the occupational areas of work, leisure and self care. Although this model has generated a great deal of interest in the UK since the early 1980s, it should be remembered that it is only one of a large number of models in use in the USA, and it is not without its critics. Nor is it widely in use in the UK, partly because of its apparent complexity when first encountered, and partly because practice relies substantially on the battery of related assessments which are not readily available in the UK. None the less, the model has been seminal and provoked a much greater interest in model building and professional philosophy than existed previously.

The adaptation through occupations model developed by Kathleen Reed is more wide ranging than the model of human occupation. It was first presented in *Concepts of Occupational Therapy* (Reed & Sanderson 1980). It describes the individual as functioning within the biopsychological, physical and sociocultural environments, continually adapting and providing for his/her needs by means of occupational behaviour in the areas of leisure, self maintenance and productivity. It defines areas of skill with which the occupational therapist should be concerned, and specfies the assumptions which lie at the heart of the practice of OT. This model is readily related to UK practice and has been implemented in a number of areas.

The adaptive skills model. Following Finlay (1988) I have used this title as a shorthand term to describe the ideas developed by Anne Cronin Mosey. Mosey has written several books on the theory and practice of OT since the late 1960s (Mosey 1968, 1973, 1981, 1986) as well as numerous papers, and it is not surprising that her work shows both considerable development and therefore some inevitable inconsistency over that period of time. All her work is written in the context of psychiatry.

In *Recapitulation of Ontogenesis* (1968), Mosey views learnt skills (especially psychosocial ones) and developmental adaptation as the keys to individual function. Her structured treatment process relates to the educational/developmental models and is humanist in outlook, but it also uses elements from behaviourism, and this has been criticized as inconsistent (Reed 1984). However, the inconsistency is resolved if the model is also viewed as primarily a problem solving system.

Her latest publication, *Psychosocial Components of Occupational Therapy*, is an evolution from and synthesis of her previous thinking, and includes analytical, acquisitional (behavioural) and developmental frames of reference. Her theories do not appear to be widely implemented in Britain.

THE MODEL OF HUMAN OCCUPATION
(*Gary Kielhofner*)

This model may, at first sight, seem somewhat obscure due to the unfamilar language and the detailed complexity of its structure. Once 'translated', the concepts become more familiar. Any attempt at summarizing the model in a few pages risks being reductionist — which is very much out of keeping with the scope and philosophy of the model.

Origins of the model

Kielhofner has drawn together a number of different areas of knowledge and a basic familiarity with these theories and their terminology is helpful. Some of the most significant are summarized. (Authorities which he quotes as sources are given in square brackets.)

Systems theory. He uses systems language — throughput, input, output — to describe the human system, and distinguishes between 'open system thinking' (i.e. the organismic view of a person continuously changing and interacting with the environment) and 'closed system thinking' (i.e. the mechanistic view of a system running unchangingly following a fixed pattern). [Allport]

Ecology: the study of an organism across time in relation to its environment; also man/environment interaction and open systems.

Cognitive psychology. The individual's abilities to perceive and process information and to organize time and tasks are important. The temporal dimension is particularly emphasized. [Bruner, an educational psychologist, is quoted and there are echoes of Lewin's concepts of life space/psychological environment; vectors trajectory; temporal orientation; search for meaning.]

Developmental psychology. These ideas include development over time (ontogenesis); continual change and growth; developing cognition in an hierarchical manner; exploration and mastery. [Piaget; Bruner]

Humanism. The model strongly emphasizes personal causation; self-actualization; choice; primacy of volition; making of meaning. [Rogers; Maslow; Lewin]

Existentialism: a philosophy which deals with the importance of the individual and individual perceptions of existence, and choices in life [Sartre]. However Kielhofner rejects the essential meaninglessness of life proposed by this philosophy.

OT theory. Kielhofner was a student of Mary Reilly and was greatly influenced by her. She developed a framework of ideas around the concept of 'occupational behaviour' during the 1960s. The model is strongly centred around human occupations.

The human open system

The model proposes that a human being should be viewed as an open system. Such a system encompasses the interrelated functions of mind/body/environment. Behaviour is purposeful (teleological), meaningful and exceeds utilitarian requirement. The system is capable of introspection and must be studied from a phenomenological perspective.

An open system operates as a hierarchy — in which all parts influence each other, but higher order functions govern the lower, and lower constrain the higher. The system operates by a process of circularity into, through and out of it.

Output, or the product of the system, is *occupational behaviour,* which is classified as work, daily living tasks, leisure or play. Output is either adaptive or maladaptive (functional or dysfunctional).

Input (intake) to the system comes from the environment; it includes information from the surrounding people, events and objects.

Throughput processes the input, organizing information, making predictions on which to base action and decisions on further action or output.

Feedback returns information to the system about the performance and consequences of action, both from the input and from the monitoring of internal processes, e.g. how one feels about what one has done.

The structure of the model

The model of human occupation is an attempt at conceptualizing the underlying dynamics of human behaviour. It arranges three subsystems in a hierarchy. An event anywhere in the system affects the whole system — it 'resonates' through it. One must therefore consider the system as an indivisible, interrelated whole, and not attempt to reduce it to its parts. The elements of the system combine to produce (or fail to produce) effective occupational behaviour. Each subsystem contains subsections.

The three subsystems can be summarized as:

VOLITION = WILL
(The mechanisms whereby we choose what to do.)

HABITUATION = ROLES AND RULES
(The basic structures with which we organize our lives.)

PERFORMANCE = SKILLS
(The means by which we carry out occupational behaviour.)

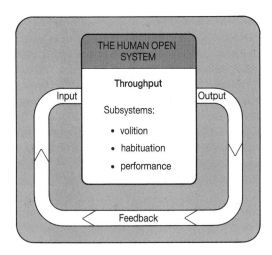

Fig. 4.1 The model of human occupation. (Reproduced with permission from Creek J 1990 Occupational Therapy and Mental Health. Churchill Livingstone, Edinburgh.)

Subsystems of the model of human occupation	
Volition	*(Will)*
● Personal causation	(Control; effectiveness)
● Values	(Standards; meaningfulness)
● Interests	(Liking and doing)
Habituation	*(Roles & rules)*
● Roles	(Owning various roles)
● Habits	(Organization; flexibility)
Performance	*(Skill)*
● Skills	(Interpersonal; process; motor; perceptual)

The volitional subsystem

Personal causation

This is concerned with whether the individual perceives himself as a competent or incompetent actor in the world. It involves:

Internal/external control. To what extent does the individual see himself as in control (an 'Origin') or controlled by others/events (a 'Pawn')?

Belief in skill. Does the individual see himself as able to perform competently and with the capacity to achieve mastery?

Expectancy of success/failure. What results of action are anticipated, as a result of past experiences?

Values

These determine whether or not an individual will engage in an occupation. Values are related to:

Temporal orientation — orientation towards past/present/future; attitudes to the use of time.

Meaningfulness of activities — only activities meaningful to the individual will provide self-satisfaction; meaningless activities are either avoided, or produce negative feelings.

Occupational goals — things one chooses to do for a reason.

Personal standards — which decide whether one is satisfied with results and likely to engage in the activity again.

Interests

Discrimination — what things interest the individual?

Pattern — are interests widely or narrowly based?

Potency — how much are interests actually pursued; how much time is given to each?

The habituation subsystem

In order to perform occupations, skills must be assembled into processes and processes organized into routines. Occupational performance implies the adoption of a variety of life roles, and the individual has to recognize these and adapt behaviour accordingly.

Roles — the variety of roles the individual has; roles change throughout life.

Perceived incumbency — the person must view him/herself as 'owning' the role.

Internalized obligations — roles carry with them obligations which must be understood and accepted.

Role balance — the mixture of roles in areas of work/play/self care should be balanced and appropriate for age.

Habits — the automated processes and routines which 'oil the wheels' and help us to organize our lives.

Degree of organization — the ability to organize time, effort, etc.

Social appropriateness — the degree to which habits are acceptable to others in the appropriate cultural context.

Rigidity and flexibility — the degree to which a person can adapt and alter.

The performance subsystem

This enables the individual competently to carry out tasks, processes and interactions.

Skills — the abilities which are needed for competent task performance.

Perceptual-motor skills — sensory and musculoskeletal.

Process skills — cognitive and sequencing skills.

Communication/interpersonal skills — required for relationships.

Skills have three subcomponents:
Symbolic — manipulation of concepts;
Neurological — perceptual/sensory interpretation and control;
Musculoskeletal — movements.

> Volition is the primary directing force. How does individual experience affect this subsystem? What are the implications of this for therapy?

Other significant concepts

Adaptive (benign) or maladaptive (vicious) cycles

Peoples' behaviour is influenced by their experiences of success or otherwise. Although this theory uses terms derived from operant conditioning, Kielhofner takes a cognitive/humanist, not a behaviourist, view of the following process. You strive for self-actualization; your experience of success in controlling your life, performing occupations and roles which you value and in exploring and mastering the environment, gains you a reinforced feeling of competence. You therefore enjoy life and continue to achieve, explore and control. In this you are in an *adaptive cycle*.

However, opposite experiences have the reverse effect; thus personal failure, perceptions of not being in control, not being competent, becoming damaged and unable to function and continually doing valueless things, reinforces the feeling that you can do nothing, and you therefore attempt less and less, and become less and less satisfied with life. You are then in a *maladaptive cycle*.

To help a client break out of a maladaptive cycle, the therapist must provide reinforcing experiences of control, competence, enjoyment and success.

An open system, being alive and reactive, is seen as travelling, being on a path of development — a *trajectory* — never static, always in the process of becoming — either better or worse. The system seeks harmony, i.e. balance, and seeks to repair disharmony, i.e. damage. These processes impart movement and direction to the system. Changes in any part of the system *resonate*, i.e. reverberate through the system affecting all other parts.

Environmental press

Kielhofner stresses the importance of the effect of the environment on the individual: his ideas here have been developed further by Barris (1982). The environment contains things which are capable of arousing us and promoting action; these include objects, tasks, social groups and cultural pressures. A degree of novelty and stimulation is pleasurable and promotes exploration and mastery. People generally perform well in such conditions.

Too much press, e.g. excessive novelty, over-stimulation or being bombarded by the demands of an environment, results in stress, anxiety, uncertainty, helplessness, frustration, anger, over-arousal and inability to cope ('flight or fight' responses). People fail to perform in such environments. Too little press results in apathy, withdrawal and disinterest, in which circumstances people also fail to perform well.

A continuum of function and dysfunction

Functional occupational behaviour is achieved through *exploration* ('curious investigation in a safe environment to discover potentials for action and properties of the environment'), which leads to *competence* ('striving to be adequate to the demands of a situation') and *achievement* ('striving to maintain and enhance standards of performance').

Dysfunction runs from *inefficiency* ('reduction or interference with performance, resulting in disatisfaction') to *incompetence* (inability to routinely and adequately perform'), and finally *helplessness* ('total or near-total disruption of performance').

In restoring function, the patient may need to be taken through the stages of safe exploration until competence is achieved, and will then need to experience competent behaviour over a period of time in order to gain a sense of achievement.

Value of productive occupations

Some models value the process more highly than the product, which may almost become irrelevant. In this model, the value and meaning of the product to the patient is seen as highly relevant and therapeutic, operating as it does directly on the volitional subsystem.

Standardized assessments

Probably because of his background in psychology, Kielhofner is committed to using standardized instruments to assess aspects of function within the terms of his model. He gives examples

---

Application of the model

General approach:

- Assess — identify problems.
- Intervene at highest level — solve problems. Or, if higher level intervention is impractical, intervene at a lower level, in order to create resonances through the system, affecting the problem area.
- The system is strongly affected by feedback from the results of actions on the environment, therefore altering the feedback by changing the environment or the nature of the patient's perceptions of his/her effect on it will alter the throughput and therefore the output of the system.
- Provide exploration as a means to attain competence and achievement.

Questions posed by the model of human occupation

Volition

1 What does the patient most want, and why does she want it?
2 How does the patient perceive control in her life?
3 What does she like to do, and what is the pattern of her occupations? Is this balanced?
4 Does she believe she is skilled and able to achieve?

Habituation

5 What roles has she had/does she have and will she perform?
6 What roles does she perceive herself as owning, and what obligations does she believe these place on her?
7 How well organized is her use of time?
8 Does she have adaptive, acceptable habits?
9 Is she rigid, or flexible and able to adapt?

Performance

10 How skilled is she in all aspects of work, leisure and self care?
11 What is her level of cognitive perceptual and physical functioning in relation to occupations?
12 Are there any skills deficits — cognitive, perceptual, motor, sensory, interpersonal?

in his book. It is not, in fact, possible to work effectively within this model without assessing aspects such as perceptions of control and competence; use of time; values; interests.

I interpret the basic treatment principles of the model as asking a sequence of questions (see p. 62). Interventions are then directed towards solving the perceived problems within the sturcture of the hierarchy.

Summary of the model of human occupation

Metamodel: Organismic.

Origin of problem: Described within the language of the model as a dysfunction in volition, habituation or performance; or input, throughput, feedback or output.

Primary assumptions
- The human organism can be described as an open system.
- Occupations are central to human experience, survival and satisfaction.
- Occupational areas of work, self care and play (leisure) evolve and change throughout the individual's life.
- Occupational performance results from the interaction of a hierarchy composed of volition, habituation and performance.
- People seek to explore and master their environments.
- The individual's perceptions of feedback from the environment are crucial in directing further output of adaptive *Holistic* occupational performance.

Terminology: Patient/client; therapist; intervention/ treatment; adaption/maladaption; function/ dysfunction; specific terminology of model (see previous notes).

Patient/therapist relationship: Therapist assesses problem and proposes problem solving intervention; patient cooperates or may direct.

Examples of applications: There appears to be no restriction on application: the literature deals with both psychiatric and physical dysfunction, and learning disorders. All age groups are covered. However, the model is perhaps least

Not age or dx specific.

appropriate for straightforward physical cases, where a biomechanical approach will suffice, and the use of the model would be time consuming and unwieldly.

Examples of techniques: The model is strongly based on the application of occupations. Within that framework, anything drawn from an organismic approach may be used, particularly cognitive and developmentally based techniques.

Evaluation of outcome: The patient shows improvement in defined deficits affecting the volition, habituation or performance subsystems, resulting in increased competence and achievement in occupational behaviour.

Advantages: A coherent set of theories is presented to direct the sequence and priorities of interventions. Psychological aspects of physical dysfunction are recognized. The model is widely applicable to all types of patients and may be particularly useful for unravelling complex problems. Patient motivation is regarded as crucial. It introduces the concepts of benign and vicious cycles, and environmental press. Standardized assessments are used.

Disadvantages: The model is founded on an unproven and, as yet, relatively unresearched hypothesis about the basis of human behaviour. The concepts and language are complex. If dealing with a simple problem, use of the whole process may be unwieldly — a 'sledgehammer to crack a nut'. The assessment process is thorough, but lengthy; as a result, a problem may be well identified but a full programme may be overly time consuming to implement. Access to appropriate assessment instruments is required. The model is biased towards volitional explanations of dysfunction, rather than physiological ones. Behavioural and analytical techniques are not compatible with the philosophy of the model.

NOTE: Dr Keilhofner's model is, at the time of publication, subject to evolution. Students are advised to watch for the publication of new material which may change the content of the model.

SUGGESTED READING

Barris R 1982 Environmental interactions: an extension of the model of human occupation. American Journal of Occupational Therapy 36 (10)

Burton J 1989 The model of human occupation and occupational therapy practice with elderly patients, Part 1: Characteristics of aging; Part 2: Application. British Journal of Occupational Therapy 52 6 215–222

Hopkins H L, Smith H D (eds) 1988 Willard & Spackman's occupational therapy. Lippincott, Philadelphia

Kielhofner G, Burke J P 1980 A model of human occupation, part 1. Conceptual framework and content. American Journal of Occupational Therapy 34 (9): 572–581

Kielhofner G 1980 A model of human occupation, part 2. Ontogenesis from the perspective of temporal adaptation. American Journal of Occupational Therapy 34 (10): 657–663

Kielhofner G 1980 A model of human occupation, part 3. Benign and vicious cycles. American Journal of Occupational Therapy 34 (11): 731–737

Kielhofner G, Burke J P, Igi C H 1980 A model of human occupation, part 4. Assessment and intervention. American Journal of Occupational Therapy 34 (12): 777–778

Kielhofner G, Nicol M 1989 The model of human occupation: a developing conceptual tool for clinicians. British Journal of Occupational Therapy 52:6 210–214

Kielhofner G (ed) 1985 A model of human occupations. Williams & Wilkins, Baltimore

Kielhofner G 1988 The model of human occupation workbook. Workshops, London, Edinburgh, York

Reed K L 1984 Models of practice in occupational therapy. Williams & Wilkins, Baltimore (ch 9)

ADAPTATION THROUGH OCCUPATION

(Kathlyn Reed)

Kathlyn Reed's model, like Kielhofner's, is still evolving, and you should try to read her recent description of it (Reed 1984) as well as her original presentation (Sanderson & Reed 1980). The model is based on problem solving and shares with the model of human occupation a strongly humanist approach, emphasizing autonomy (functional independence), actualization (self-satisfaction) and

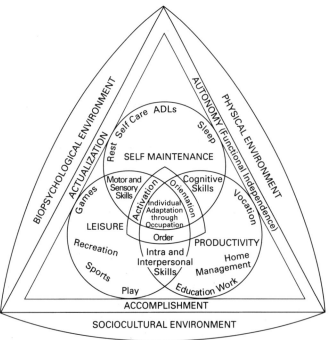

Fig. 4.2 Adaptation through occupation model. (Reproduced from Reed K L 1984 Models of practice in occupational therapy, Williams & Wilkins, Baltimore.)

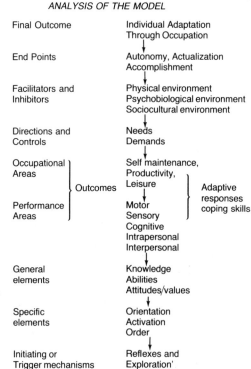

ANALYSIS OF THE MODEL

Final Outcome	Individual Adaptation Through Occupation
End Points	Autonomy, Actualization Accomplishment
Facilitators and Inhibitors	Physical environment Psychobiological environment Sociocultural environment
Directions and Controls	Needs Demands
Occupational Areas	Self maintenance, Productivity, Leisure
Performance Areas	Motor Sensory Cognitive Intrapersonal Interpersonal
General elements	Knowledge Abilities Attitudes/values
Specific elements	Orientation Activation Order
Initiating or Trigger mechanisms	Reflexes and Exploration'

(Occupational Areas and Performance Areas bracketed together as *Outcomes*; Self maintenance/Productivity/Leisure and Motor/Sensory/Cognitive/Intrapersonal/Interpersonal bracketed together as *Adaptive responses coping skills*)

accomplishment (doing required things well), and a focus on occupations as fundamental to human existence and health. The individual is seen as an interactive open system, but without the specific hierarchy of concepts associated with the human occupations model. The model also echoes Mosey's strongly developmental frame of reference and her emphasis on learning and adapting. Participation in occupations and alterations of the environment are both seen as powerful mechanisms for change.

Reed is particularly concerned to identify the unique processes, concepts, techniques, concerns, assumptions and outcomes of OT. She feels it important to focus on 'wellness' not medical model 'illness'. She has a highly structured view of the process and application of occupational therapy, stressing that occupations can be therapeutic because they are the natural vehicles for normal development and adaptation and for the primary learning of skills. Skill assessment, development and retraining is seen as a main concern of occupational therapists. The therapist can help the individual to develop adaptive responses through participation in occupations.

The environment

Reed proposes that occupational performance is influenced by the environmental context and content, which may enhance or impede learning and performance. She suggests that analysis of the environment by the therapist is a significant therapeutic tool in identifying the causes of maladaptation and in enhancing and facilitating adaptive performance. The environment can be subdivided into:

- *Physical environment:* inanimate, non-human and natural aspects.
- *Biopsychological environment:* the individual self — the human being. (The idea of the body/mind of the person being part of the environment is interesting — it can be connected with Lewin's 'life space'.)
- *Sociocultural environment:* people and their cultures, attitudes, values and means of organization.

Occupations

These can be divided contextually into:

- *Self-maintenence*
- *Productivity*
- *Leisure*

and into component *tasks* (but each occupation is performed as a gestalt).

Occupations have five *performance areas*. Each performance area requires the use of abilities and *skills* which are classified as :

- *Motor*
- *Sensory*
- *Cognitive*
- *Interpersonal* (between self and others)
- *Intrapersonal* (within self: identity, emotions, coping skills)

For assessment of these skills, Reed uses headings derived from a modification of Gagné's (1977) eight stages of learning, including skill development, chained behaviour, information processing and problem solving.

The performance of occupations requires three *general elements* which are learnt:

- *Knowledge*
- *Abilities*
- *Attitudes/values*

There are also three specific elements related to occupational therapy:

- *Orientation* (to time, place and person)
- *Order* (pattern and direction)
- *Activation* (ability to move and think)

Occupational adaptation and adjustment

The goal of the individual is life-satisfaction through occupational adaptation. Occupations should enable the person to relate to the environment and to meet needs by balanced performance within the areas of productivity, self-maintenence and leisure. Occupations have associated standards, roles and meaning for the individual. Occupational behaviour is either adaptive or mal/nonadapative.

Adaptive behaviour — uses skills to achieve balanced experience of occupations consistent with social norms and self-satisfaction.

Maladaptive behaviour — is unsuccessful and/or unacceptable to the individual or society.

Nonadaptive behaviour — fails to produce effective results, but is not unacceptable.

Occupational dysfunction — problems in planning and/or performing an occupation or in evaluating feedback of results.

Therapeutic occupations — should be one or more of the following: meaningful; purposeful; goal directed; challenging. Reed offers an extended discussion of the individual and subjective nature of meaning in terms of occupational performance, and emphasizes the essentially purposeful nature of therapeutic activities.

Outcomes

Reed states outcomes of occupational therapy clearly and concisely, and these are best quoted as written:

1 The person will be able to perform or have performed those occupations which meet the individual's needs and are acceptable to the person and society.
2 The person will have the necessary performance skills which compose the occupations in the individual's repertoire of self-maintenance, productivity and leisure.
3 The person will have a balance of occupations such that actualization, autonomy and achievement are attained to a maximum degree of adaptation.
4 The person will be able to adapt to the environment or cause the environment to adapt to the individual.
5 The person will be able to meet both deficiency needs and growth needs.
6 Where the person is unable to perform skills independently, assistive devices or equipment or other environmental adjustments may be used.

(Reed 1984)

Summary of adaptation through occupation

Metamodel: Organismic; humanist/developmental/educational.

Origin of problem: The patient shows dysfunctional, maladaptive or nonadaptive performance; the patient is unable to use a skill, does not use it, has not developed it or has never acquired it.

Primary assumptions

- A person changes, adapts, achieves satisfaction by means of occupational performance within physical and sociocultural environments.
- Occupational performance consists of learnt skills.
- Training in skills, engagement in occupations and/or modification of the environment can result in restoration of adaptive performance.

Terminology: Patient; therapist; therapy; function/dysfunction; adaptation/maladaptation; description of environment, occupations, tasks, skills within terms of the model.

Patient/therapist relationship: Therapist assesses, proposes or negotiates intervention; patient co-operates or may direct.

Examples of applications: Any person who, for whatever cause:

a. has failed to develop occupational skills in any of the three areas;
b. has temporary or permanent loss of occupational skills;
c. whose performance of occupational skills requires non-routine modification;
d. is at risk of losing occupational skills.

(Sanderson & Reed 1980)

Examples of techniques: Anything appropriate to the problem. Since the model is strongly organismic, techniques should be compatible; however, modified behaviourist techniques may be appropriate, and biomechanical ones are certainly suggested. Analytical techniques seem less relevant since they are not compatible with a strongly humanist approach and the model does not pay much attention to unconscious mechanisms.

Advantages: A flexible, practical, holistic, client centred, problem solving approach; strong, coherent presentation of OT theory; compatible with a wide range of techniques; focuses on 'wellness' not 'illness'.

Disadvantages: Few obvious ones. It disregards unconscious motivations and says little about group processes which are not based on goal directed occupations.

SUGGESTED READING

Gagné R M 1977 The conditions of learning and theory of instruction, 3rd edn. Holt Saunders, New York

Sanderson S, Reed K L 1980 Concepts of occupational therapy. Williams & Wilkins, Baltimore

Reed K L 1984 Models of practice in occupational therapy. Williams & Wilkins, Baltimore

ADAPTIVE SKILLS
(Anne Cronin Mosey)

In contrast to the previous generic models, that proposed by Anne Cronin Mosey is primarily related to psychiatric practice. Her ideas were first developed during the late 1960s and early 70s, but her recent work provides a synthesis of previous ideas. Like Reed, she views occupational therapy as being principally concerned with skills and adaptation, and she has strong views about the legitimate tools and concerns of the profession. Like Kielhofner, she uses the systems language of input, throughput, output and feedback to describe the OT process. She does not herself describe her ideas as a 'model' since she reserves that term for the higher level which other writers call a paradigm, a term she rejects as inapplicable to OT (Mosey 1981). In terms of organization and integration, however, it clearly compares with other models described in this book.

Her model is aimed at dealing with problems in psychosocial function. She explains these as either a learned maladaptive response or a lack of skill, affecting task planning and performance, interactions or ability to identify and satisfy needs.

In this context she lists four *performance components*:

- *Sensory integration*
- *Cognitive function*
- *Psychological function*
- *Social interaction.*

These four components are used in five areas of occupational performance:

- *Family interactions*
- *Activities of daily living*
- *School/work*
- *Play/leisure/recreation*
- *Temporal adaptation.*

Occupational performance takes place in the context of the environment, which can be divided into *cultural environment*, *social environment* and *physical environment*.

Three frames of reference (Mosey 1970, 1986)

These are proposed for use in psychiatric occupational therapy. All three frames of reference deal with the use of activities as vehicles for skill or role development.

The *analytical frame of reference* is described as being appropriate when dealing with a client whose life situation involves difficulties with 'universal issues'. These are listed as: reality; trust; intimacy; adequacy; dependence/independence; sexuality; aggression. Mosey's interpretation of the analytical approach is eclectic, but appears to be based more on object relations theories than Freudian ones.

The *acquisitional frame of reference* has a

cognitive/behavioural base, and deals mainly with the acquisition of interpersonal skills and roles.

In *recapitulation of ontogenesis*, Mosey uses a developmental/humanist frame of reference, but links this with elements of cognitive and social learning theory. She identifies six (originally seven: drive-object skill was removed from later lists) *adaptive skills*. These skills are acquired sequentially and are universal. They include the following:

Perceptual motor skill: The ability to receive, select, combine and coordinate vestibular, proprioceptive and tactile information for functional use.

Cognitive skill: The ability to perceive, represent and organize sensory information for the purpose of thinking and problem solving.

Dyadic interaction skill: The ability to participate in a variety of dyadic relationships.

Group interaction skill: The ability to engage in a variety of primary groups.

Self identity skill: The ability to perceive the self as a relatively autonomous, holistic and acceptable person who has permanence and continuity over time.

Sexual identity skill: The ability to perceive one's sexual nature as good and to participate in a relatively long term sexual relationship that is oriented to the mutual satisfaction of sexual needs.

(Mosey 1986)

(Note: This list is taken from Mosey's most recent publication, and differs in some small but significant aspects from her previous definitions.)

These adaptive skills are composed of *adaptive subskills* which in turn are composed of *skill components*. Perhaps the most interesting and potentially useful part of the model is the analysis of each of the six skills as a developmental sequence, linked to chronological developmental stages in which each skill evolves in complexity and adaptive potential. An assessment of the level of function therefore enables one to determine a developmental age or level for the individual in each skill. This enables activities and interactions to be selected at the correct level so that early

skills can be learnt or regained before later ones and the correct developmental sequence is retained. (This is similar to the approach of Allen (1985), who proposes a cognitive/developmental system using very well structured activities aimed at identified levels.)

Assessments and interventions are related to each of these areas, depending on the type of dysfunction, and a range of standardized tests is proposed. In common with Reed and Kielhofner, Mosey quotes Reilly and emphasizes the use of activity, both for individuals and structured groups. Experiential learning through activity, interactions and group work is seen as the means of producing adaptive responses or improving skills.

Like Reed, she is concerned with 'wellness' rather than 'illness' and suggests a list of 'health needs' which a therapist should be aware of and should attempt to meet through occupational therapy programmes. Because her base is in psychiatric practice, the purpose of this list seems largely to be the fostering of anti-institutionalized relationships and programmes.

This list has similarities with Maslow's heirarchy of needs, and includes:

Health needs

Psychophysical needs (physiological, environmental)
Temporal balance and regularity (varied pattern of occupations and timing)
Safety (physical and emotional)
Love and acceptance (client/therapist relationship)
Group association (sharing)
Mastery (successful participation in activity)
Esteem (a valued, rewarding role)
Sexual needs (recognizing needs; enabling needs to be met)
Pleasure (client's individual definition)
Self-actualization (meaningful activities and relationships)

Mosey presents a detailed and densely argued account of occupational therapy which cannot be encapsulated in a few pages. Her ideas are pragmatic and those who find them interesting are recommended to try to obtain her more recent publications, which are unfortunately not easy to acquire in the UK. (Mosey does not give a visual representation of her ideas, and it would be presumptuous to invent one).

Summary of the adaptative skills model

Metamodel: Organismic. (Reed criticises the model as philosophically inconsistent because it combines deterministic elements from behaviourism and analytical theory with developmental/humanist theories. Whilst Mosey does discuss the three frames of reference, she does not imply simultaneous use, but rather sees these as alternatives, based on a pragmatic, problem solving approach to a client's needs. The model remains basically holistic.)

Origin of problem: Lack of adaptive skills due to incorrect or incomplete learning; disrupted maturation or incomplete developmental sequence; environmental stress; physical or psychological abnormality.

Primary assumptions

- Adaptive skills are required for the satisfactory performance of activities and interactions.
- Adaptive skills are learnt, and can be trained or regained in a developmental sequence.
- Therapeutic activities and interventions should be pitched to match the initial developmental level of the individual and

progressed as the individual masters each stage.

Terminology: Client/patient; therapist; therapy; adaptive skills; function/dysfunction; adaption/maladaption.

Patient/therapist relationship: Therapist assesses and provides prescribed intervention; patient cooperates and may assist with goal setting. The value of the development of a trusting, caring relationship between client and therapist, and the therapist's 'conscious use of self' as a therapeutic tool is emphasized.

Examples of applications: Psychiatric disorders, both acute and long term. People who have symptoms of psychosocial dysfunction.

Examples of techniques: These are related to the six adaptive skills and may include: activities to promote sensory integration; cognitive activities; perceptual activities; dyadic and group interactions and activities; activities to enhance self image and identity; sexual counselling and interactive role play; behavioural learning techniques; social modelling.

Advantages: Recognizes that progress cannot be achieved if the individual has not reached the required developmental level — identifies level and assists correct choice of activities in correct sequence. Useful for individuals functioning at a low level.

Disadvantages: The strongly psychosocial emphasis leads to restricted applicablity in physical settings.

SUGGESTED READING

Mosey A C 1968 Recapitulation of ontogenesis: a theory for the practice of occupational therapy. American Journal of Occupational Therapy 22: (5)
Mosey A C 1970 Three frames of reference for mental health. Slack, New Jersey
Mosey A C 1973 Activities therapy. Raven Press, New York

Mosey A C 1981 Occupational therapy: configuration of a profession. Raven Press, New York
Mosey A C 1986 Psychosocial components of occupational therapy. Raven Press, New York
Reed K L 1984 Models of practice in occupational therapy. Williams & Wilkins, Baltimore

5

Core skills

WHAT ARE CORE SKILLS AND WHY ARE THEY IMPORTANT?

After reviewing a selection of contrasting and sometimes conflicting theoretical structures, the reader may well be left wondering whether it is possible to describe a central, generic core of professional practice in occupational therapy. This is not a new question, nor is there a simple answer.

As this study guide illustrates, occupational therapists use different approaches and techniques depending on the speciality and location in which each therapist works, and his/her experience. There may appear to be little in common between the therapist who assesses the home for the provision of an adapted ground floor extension, the one who takes a session of psychodrama and the one who rehabilitates a patient's hand function following a severe crush injury.

What, then, is occupational therapy and how does its practice differ from that of similar professions? Is practice purely contextual and a matter of individual style? Good multidisciplinary teamwork frequently encourages the blurring of professional boundaries — it matters less *who* does it, than that it is done effectively. But if it does not matter, and if anyone can do the job, who needs the therapist?

The standard definition of occupational therapy used by the World Federation of Occupational Therapists is, 'The treatment of physical and psychiatric conditions through specific selected activities in order to help people to reach their maximum level of function in all aspects of daily life'. Whilst this has the virtue of brevity, inevitably it cannot encapsulate the full spectrum of current OT practice; it does not fit comfortably with the extending field of practice in the community, nor can it give any but the most generalized indication of what the practitioner does. There are several other definitions, all longer, and all subject to criticism.

'What do *we* do that is different?' is a central question for any profession. If the question is not answered for occupational therapy, it becomes difficult to define the body of knowledge or the standard of skill which students must acquire if they are to become competent practitioners. It is also difficult to define and defend service provision, to set and maintain standards, to ensure quality, or to ensure that occupational therapists' skills are used to best effect, which is of increasing importance when therapists are in short supply.

For these reasons, there has been a recent increase in interest, both from the profession and its managers, in the process of identifying and describing core skills. This process is not without its dangers. If carried to extremes, it can become reductive, and therapy may come to be regarded as a mechanistic process more at a technician's level than that of a professional practitioner. As discussed in the keynote address at the World Federation of Occupational Therapists' Congress in 1990 (Barnitt 1990), the attempt to define the knowledge, skills and attitudes which form the structure of the profession may lead us towards adopting standardized practices and formulae which actually inhibit thinking and dynamic professional development. Our core skills must, somehow, encompass the nebulous aspects of professional judgement, problem solving and research, as well as the more readily assessed aspects of 'hands on' therapeutic knowledge and skill.

A core skill may be defined as one of the essential elements of generic professional practice, the use of which remains relatively constant, although adapted by the selection of therapeutic models or frames of reference.

It is doubtful whether there is currently a sufficient consensus within the profession over what constitutes legitimate and 'illegitimate' professional practice for a single list of core skills to be ac-

> **Q** Before going any further, write down your own list of occupational therapy core skills — the things which are essential for effective practice. When you have compiled your list, divide the skills listed into those which *only* occupational therapists use, or use in a unique way, and those which other medical or paramedical professions use. If you can, compare your list with someone else's — do they differ? How, and why?

cepted. All such analysis is artificial; in practice, therapy operates as a gestalt. However, the more people criticise the available lists and attempt new ones, the sooner the profession will evolve an accepted core.

The literature is unhelpful. Whilst the occupational therapy process is often described, if you look at this critically, it does not differ substantially from the treatment process used by any similar profession. It is actually the basic problem solving process:

- gain information
- define the problem
- set objectives
- plan action
- implement
- review.

As shown by Fig. 5.1, which clearly illustrates the circular nature of the process, it would be possible to remove the central words 'occupational therapy' and then substitute the name of any similar profession — physiotherapy, speech therapy, psychology or nursing.

Most attempts at defining the skills required to practise occupational therapy are made, consciously or unwittingly, from the perspective of the writer's speciality and preferred structure. These definitions bring with them specific skills and emphasize specific aspects. Such definitions often fail to distinguish between those elements which are generic and those which are derived from the particular structure and circumstances.

Mosey, for example, states that 'a profession is characterized by a description of six elements: the profession's philosophical assumptions, ethical code, body of knowledge, domain of concern, nature of and principles for sequencing the various

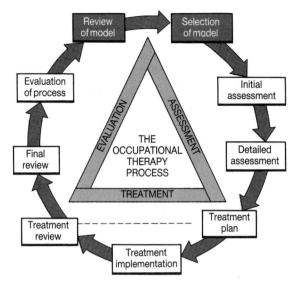

Fig. 5.1 The OT process. (Reproduced with permission from Creek J 1990 Occupational Therapy and Mental Health. Churchill Livingstone, Edinburgh.)

aspects of practice, and the profession's legitimate tools' (Mosey 1986).

In the case of occupational therapy, with its broad knowledge and skill base, there may well be considerable overlap between it and similar professions allied to medicine in all but two of these areas: the domain of concern — which Mosey describes as occupational performance — and the legitimate tools of the profession. These are listed as 'the non-human environment, conscious use of self, the teaching-learning process, purposeful activity, activity groups, and activity analysis and synthesis.' This list is useful in that it is clearly an 'OT list' and no one else's, but it is related to Mosey's own perception of the OT process as used in the context of psychosocial practice.

The following analysis is my attempt at the production of a generic list of core skills, to which can be added the skills required when working within specific approaches. The word *skill* has been used as a convenient shorthand to mean 'a learnt ability and applied knowledge used to achieve a task to a definable standard of competence'. The word 'competency' can be substituted, but has been avoided. (I have already noted that theorists cannot escape from their own preconceptions and bias — I am no exception.)

CLASSIFICATION OF CORE SKILLS

Core skills may be subdivided into three groups:

- **Managerial skills**
- **Interactive skills**
- **Therapeutic skills.**

These, in turn, may be seen as falling into one of three groups:

Generic core skills: those skills which are common to the treatment process employed by occupational therapists and other similar health care professions. OTs will put their own professional slant on these skills, but they are not radically changed when used by different professions, and at the level of basic training much of the knowledge base could be shared.

Primary core skills: those managerial, interactive and therapeutic skills which are specific to occupational therapy or which occupational therapists use in a way which is particular to the profession.

Secondary core skills. In addition to the generic and primary core skills, each OT approach generates the need for a specific focus and the requirement that particular therapeutic or interactive skills be developed, or others discarded. Some of these skills are acquired at basic level, at least in outline, but others develop with experience and would only be found in senior practitioners. These will not be listed here: examples can be found in the summary of techniques used in each approach. Also included in this category are the advanced managerial skills required by senior practitioners.

GENERIC CORE SKILLS
Managerial skills

Organizational skills, e.g. independent management of self and own resources; routine administration; appointments systems; planning delivery of services; delegating work to assistants; monitoring workload.

Financial skills, e.g. effective, efficient and economical provision of services; budget monitoring; ordering; stocktaking.

Recording skills, e.g. selecting relevant information; clear concise record-keeping which is comprehensible to others; using correct language and format; recording at appropriate intervals; keeping statistical records; maintaining confidentiality.

Research skills, e.g. able to undertake literature searches; construct questionnaires; understand and use simple statistics; formulate protocols for research projects; produce material for professional journals; understand basic research methodology.

Problem solving skills: use of basic problem solving methodology, e.g. strategies to define and analyse problem; select priorities for action; produce and correctly evaluate possible solutions; select optimum solution; plan and carry out action; evaluate results; redefine problem and plan new action if required.

Interactive skills

Communication skills, e.g. verbal skills; telephone skills; use of information technology; written communications; formal and informal communication methods — at professional level; with patients, carers and lay people; group and dyadic.

Supervisory skills: supervise assistants and students; coordinate the work of others.

Teaching skills, e.g. prepare and use visual aids; construct training programmes; give lectures, demonstrate and instruct students.

Basic counselling skills, e.g. non-verbal skills; listening; reflecting; cueing; prompting.

Basic group skills: awareness of the group process; being aware of a range of purposes and types of groups; be able to organize, run and monitor therapeutic groups; use of appropriate leadership styles; be able to act as co-therapist.

Therapeutic skills

Patient care skills, e.g. preservation of individual rights and dignity; awareness of individual needs; safe handling and lifting; correct choice and use of mobility aids; patient comfort and correct positioning; basic personal care, e.g. assistance with eating or use of toilet; maintenance of safe procedures and environment.

Observation skills: take account of physical appearance of patient; facial expression, posture and dress; observe external changes of medical significance, e.g. skin colour, sweating, condition of scar; observe interactions, e.g. patterns or frequency of communication, non-verbal signals; consistent relationships; note environmental content; notice hazards.

PRIMARY CORE SKILLS

Managerial skills

Therapy/intervention planning skills. Planning therapy or intervention is a managerial task in two senses: first, in 'managing' the patient or client's condition, needs or problem; and secondly, in effectively coordinating all the aspects of the therapist's personal knowledge and resources with those of others.

Therapy means treatment, which is something which involves the patient, and normally requires his/her active participation. Direct treatment is not always required and frequently there is the need for some action by the therapist which does not involve participation by the patient, hence the use of the term 'intervention'. Studies have shown that between 50% and 30% of a therapist's time may be spent in actions which are not direct 'hands on/face to face' patient treatment. For simplicity, the word therapy will be used here to cover all types of treatment and intervention.

The ability to make correct decisions about what to do, to decide on priorities, set aims and objectives, plan how these are to be achieved, and to implement these decisions efficiently are fundamental to effective therapy. Although the process is one used by others (as already noted), the basis for actions and decisions is unique to OT and requires integration of the generic core skills previously listed with primary and secondary core skills. The basic process is similar whatever approach is used, although the language, style of presentation and emphasis may change.

Evaluation skills. The maintenance of personal and professional standards is a prime responsibility of any practitioner and can only be judged in relation to the profession's specific knowledge base and primary core skills. Therapy must be evaluated to ensure that it is effective and to justify continuing or discontinuing therapy/intervention. The therapist should set standards, communicate treatment results to others, be critical of his or her own performance, monitor quality of service, seek regular supervision, evaluate and update personal knowledge, and ensure personal development.

Interactive skills

Conscious use of self. In nursing, social work or the remedial professions, the dyadic therapeutic relationship between the professional and the patient/client is of great importance. Whilst occupational therapists frequently engage in ordinary dyadic interactions, the process of occupational therapy is unique in that the relationship may be considered not as a dyad (therapist/patient) but as a *triad* (therapist/patient/occupation). The occupation is the medium whereby the interaction is enabled or explored. Whether working with an individual or with a group, the therapist's awareness of personal attributes and skills in interpersonal relationships and the sensitive and empathetic use of such attributes or skills in the context of an activity or task in order to develop a therapeutic relationship with the participant(s), and to achieve a therapeutic goal, is at the centre of the practice of occupational therapy.

The uses of this skill could include the following.

- Select and enhance features of an activity to promote specific interactions.
- Decide on the degree of direction/non-direction/leadership style.
- Use knowledge of group process appropriately.
- Allow or restrict personal spontaneity.
- Control the use of humour.
- Set limits for oneself.
- Be aware of one's own emotions and reactions: consciously use these for positive therapeutic purposes, or avoid negative effects on therapy.
- Understand one's own attitudes and prejudices and the possible effects of these on relationships; avoid being judgemental.
- Define and adhere to one's own meaning of 'professional behaviour' and 'ethics'.

- Monitor oneself and be aware of one's own needs.
- Be aware of the dangers of manipulating or dominating others.
- Give the patient appropriate reactions, e.g. praise, encouragement, consolation.
- Use confidence in oneself to give the patient confidence and trust in the treatment.
- Use initiative, imagination, creativity.

Therapeutic skills

Ability to apply factual and theoretical knowledge. OT requires a synthesis of knowledge. Although the individual components studied are shared by other professions, the precise emphasis and combination of subjects is unique to OT. Subjects studied normally include: anatomy, physiology, kinesiology, ergonomics, medicine, surgery, psychiatry, psychology, sociology, learning theory, human occupations, and the theory and practice of occupational therapy.

The assimilation and integration of this knowledge enables a therapist to:

- Comprehend the nature of traumatic or pathological processes affecting the individual.
- Comprehend the nature and causes of dysfunction in occupational performance.
- Make correct professional judgements to determine treatment aims and methods and to predict outcomes.
- Select and analyse treatment techniques, using and adapting activities as required.
- Treat the patient safely and effectively.
- Undertake research.
- Use professional literature constructively and with comprehension.
- Communicate with members of other professions.

Ability to apply technical and creative skills. Occupational therapists require a personal repertoire of practical skills and techniques at a sufficient level of competence to provide safe, flexible, imaginative and effective therapy in a range of situations and with different specialities. Skills and techniques may include knowledge of and ability to carry out/teach technical and creative processes and activities used in work, leisure or self care.

Typical skills include:

- Trade and technical skills, e.g. woodwork, metalwork, horticulture, printing, computer operation, typing, word processing.
- Craft skills, e.g. weaving, rugmaking, macrame, pottery, sewing.
- Creative and expressive skills, e.g. art, collage, drama, mime, puppetry, music, dance, creative writing.
- Domestic skills, e.g. cooking, budgeting, menu planning, domestic activities, DIY.
- Leisure skills, e.g. sport, hobbies, recreational activities, games, keep fit, outings.

Ability to apply therapeutic skills and techniques. All therapists require a basic repertoire of therapeutic skills. Whilst these will develop with experience, basic practitioners typically have some experience in a representative range of techniques.

Examples may include abilities to:

- Make and fit orthoses.
- Instruct in use of prostheses.
- Assess for, provide and train in the use of wheelchairs.
- Adapt or provide therapeutic apparatus and assistive equipment for use in activities of daily living, work or leisure.
- Make recommendations for the provision of housing adaptations for disabled people.
- Use neurodevelopmental handling, positioning and stimulation techniques (e.g. Bobath, PNF, sensori-motor techniques).
- Test and retrain perceptual-motor function.
- Use behavioural modification techniques.
- Conduct social skills training.
- Use reminiscence and reality orientation.
- Use projective techniques and media including music, art, creative writing, bibliotherapy.
- Use psychodrama, role play, guided fantasy and related techniques.

Assessment skills. Assessment of levels of performance in occupational areas, and of occupational roles and skills, comprises a large part of

OT practice. The type of assessment used and the objective of the assessment will relate to the needs of the patient and the approach within which the therapist is operating. (See Appendix 1 for a list of assessment related to different approaches).

It is acknowledged that the basic skills of assessment are also used by other professions (e.g. select what is to be assessed; select or design correct assessment methods; be objective; show good observation skills; produce consistent, accurate and, where possible, replicable results; communicate results clearly to others; be sensitive to the patient as an individual). However, in the context of OT, a crucial primary core skill is the ability to conduct assessments and to analyse the results in order to plan therapy or intervention in an area of occupational performance or dysfunction.

Asessments may be conducted within a model, or as a means of selecting one. Assessment should be recognized as a means to an end — identification of the problem; definition of a starting point for treatment/intervention; measurement of progress; evaluation of outcome — not as an end in itself.

Assessment may be formal or informal, be used once or sequentially, and can utilize a wide variety of techniques. As a generic process, assessment involves:

- information gathering;
- observation;
- measurement;
- recording;
- evaluation against a norm or outcome.

Assessment methodology. There is extensive literature concerning the structure and methods of assessment. Assessments may be:

Standardized — usually conducted following a format which has been piloted on a reasonably large sample of subjects and adjusted for inter-rater reliability. There is an explicit standard against which the results of the assessment can be judged. There are numerous standardized and validated tests on the market, particularly in the areas of cognition, intelligence, perception, personality and performance skills. Some of these would be of use to occupational therapists, but can only be purchased following special training.

Validated — objective tests following a strict format, often in a controlled environment, developed by formal research involving control groups, using researched and accepted norms of performance and tested for inter-rater reliability and statistical validity.

Informal — ad hoc, unstandardized tests. Assessments are based on subjective observation in normal environments. Many assessments are constructed by occupational therapists and whilst these employ questionnaires, checklists, grading systems and structured performance tests, few are standardized and very few properly validated — not least because this requires detailed research, large samples of patients and control groups, and because it is an extremely complex and time consuming procedure which is beyond the scope of most busy practitioners.

Single or sequential. An assessment may be a 'one off' exercise, or a sequential process where the same performance is reassessed at intervals. In either case there may be a standardized measure — or the individual's previous performance, or 'normal' performance where this is observable — which can be used as the bench-mark.

Objective or subjective. It is impossible (outside of laboratory conditions, and perhaps even then) not to be, to some extent, subjective. Some performances can be assessed with reasonable consistency against known criteria, but many can not. The criteria do not exist; the effects of environment; the therapist/patient relationship; the mood and motivation of the patient; the skills, expectations, attitudes and intentions of the observer; the well documented effects of the process of being observed on the performance of the subject — all these have the potential to alter, or at worst invalidate assessment results. In the context of OT, it may have to be accepted that intuitive methods of assessment, based on experience and professional judgement, can be valid: 'single case' studies, carefully reported, can be highly illuminating.

Assessment procedures. All assessment procedures require a basis of theoretical knowledge and practical experience and expertise. Basic methods may be used in a variety of ways, formal and in-

formal. The subject may be asked to perform an action or complete a task, or to complete a self-rating form. Alternatively, the therapist investigates or measures, whilst the subject is relatively passive.

Procedures for obtaining information. These include:

- *Interviews:* informal and unstructured, or formal and structured.
- *Questionnaires:* self-rating or administered.
- *Performance tests:* physical; cognitive; interactive.

The subject completes a task or demonstrates skill or knowledge.

- *Measurement techniques:* frequently of physical function.
- *Observation and sampling techniques:* to obtain a profile of the subject.

Procedures for collating and evaluating information. These include:

- *Rating scales:* giving a grading or numerical score.
- *Checklists:* as a structured aid to observation.
- *Record forms:* a structured aid to observation and sequential comparison.
- *Charts, grids or graphs:* a visual aid to recording and evaluating results.
- *Statistical formulae:* to evaluate significance of data.
- *Profiling:* provides a comprehensive 'picture' of the subject.

Programme planning. A prime skill of the therapist is the ability to translate aims and objectives into a programme of relevant and effective therapy. The plan specifies the methods to be used, and the conditions under which they will be used (time, place, person, etc.). Often, a plan will include a timetable and an indication of the timing of component parts. It may include details of the location of treatment, the persons involved and the techniques used. It may be very brief or highly elaborate, depending on circumstances. Either as part of the plan, or as a separate exercise, details of any occupational or environmental adaptations or grading can be included if appropriate.

As previously noted, action to be taken by the therapist is frequently required as well as, or in place of, a patient's treatment programme. For example, the therapist may need to conduct interviews, write letters or make contact with a wide range of agencies which may assist the patient, obtain equipment, plan adaptations, communicate with relatives or make visits. In the case of the community-based therapist, the latter aspects are likely to form the major part of the therapist's intervention, and may be recorded in the form of an 'Action Plan' rather than a therapeutic programme.

Analysis, adaptation and application of occupations

The analysis of occupations and their prescription as therapy are the unique skills of the occupational therapist. The analysis and prescription of occupations have two purposes:

1 To deal with problems experienced by the patient in occupations, activities and tasks related to daily living — normally classified as work, leisure and self care (ADL) — or with social roles (e.g. parent, friend, citizen).
2 The use of activities as specific therapeutic media to treat dysfunctions in the performance of occupations, interactions and roles.

Solving performance problems in occupational areas. The therapist's traditional division of occupations into work, leisure or activities of daily living must be acknowledged as artificial. In practice, the edges blur. Classification is contextual — what one person regards as a chore may be a hobby for someone else. Is housework work or self care? This method of division, and particularly the currently popular concept that life should contain an appropriate balance of the three occupational areas, is biased towards developed western-style cultures and may require considerable modification in cultures where such distinctions break down. However, it remains a convenient method of analysis.

The occupational therapist uses a variety of techniques to assess abilities and deficits, to retrain skills and to problem-solve in these occupational areas. The individuals requiring this service are frequently those who are disabled, rather than dysfunctional. Once environmental constraints are removed or methods of using residual skills to best advantage have been mastered, such individuals can become independent and contributing members of society. Therapists working in the community are likely to spend most of their time in solving performance problems and adapting environments.

Work. Any problem which prevents an individual who wishes to work from doing so is likely to have considerable social, psychological and economic consequences. The therapist may use industrial therapy, work related rehabilitation, adaptation of the workplace and preliminary vocational guidance and training to assist return to work. More complex vocational guidance and retraining is not within the scope of the therapist.

Leisure. Awareness of self actualization needs and the importance of the quality of life is increasing, and proportions of those people who are unemployed or those retired find it hard to cope with unstructured time, and need guidance. In the case of those who are unable to work due to a disability or illness, leisure may become crucial in giving purpose and meaning to life.

Activities of daily living (ADL). These activities range from those fundamental for survival — eating, keeping warm, avoiding danger, maintaining personal hygiene — to the more complex aspects of personal self care, independence, and, in some settings, basic social skills. Assessment is carried out to identify the nature and severity of the problem. A programme of practice and training is then provided in as realistic a setting as possible. Any residual disabilities which persist after a period of training are resolved by the provision of adapted equipment, environmental adaptation, or assistance for the individual.

Application of activities as therapy. The selection of a therapeutic activity requires that a balance be achieved between the needs and interests of the patient, the personal repertoire of skills possessed by the therapist and the requirements of the model or approach within which the therapist chooses to work.

Activities should be specifically selected for the individual patient with a view to a defined goal, e.g.

- assessing ability;
- meeting a need;
- solving a problem;
- providing experience;
- improving a skill;
- stimulating an interest;
- promoting independence;
- encouraging an interaction;
- stimulating exploration;
- providing opportunities for choice.

Activities may be used casually for recreation, or as pastimes; such use is perfectly valid in the right context. This may be called diversional occupation, *but it is not occupational therapy.*

Whilst engaging the patient in prescribed remedial activities remains a central professional skill, for many therapists it may play a relatively small part in their interventions, which will be concerned more with the analysis of dysfunction in occupational areas and the consequent problem solving actions, as described above.

Techniques of analysis, adaptation and application. These include:

Environmental analysis. Occupational therapists recognize that the environment can have an important beneficial or detrimental effect on the individual. Analysis of the content of the environment — at work, at home, at school, in an institution, out of doors, in a public place — may provide information on the causes of problems for the individual, explanations for behaviour or ideas, or suggestions for therapeutic modifications. The way in which environmental analysis is carried out depends on the needs of the patient and the approach within which the therapist is working as these will alter the significance of the components which are observed.

In general terms, the occupational therapist will observe and accurately record environmental content, e.g. buildings, interiors, heat, light, sound, vibration, degree of stimulation, social or cultural significance, emotional impact, and define the *environmental press* — elements which contribute to or detract from patient performance.

Environmental adaptation. The therapist will alter, remove from or add to elements of the environment, e.g. physical features of buildings, access, sound, colour, lighting level, temperature, decor, furniture, information content, in order to remove obstacles to performance or to enhance the opportunities for performance, learning or development.

Occupational analysis. This may include: contextual evaluation of whether the occupation is work, leisure or self care; examination and description of the scope of an individual's existing, past or required occupations; analysing occupations in terms of roles; analysing the socio-cultural importance or meaning of an occupation for the individual.

Activity analysis. This involves dissecting the activity into its component parts and sequence and evaluating its therapeutic potential and possible relevance to the treatment plan. Activity analysis is meaningful only in relation to defined objectives and the assessed condition of the patient. Whether the therapist is selecting a single therapeutic activity or a range of options to offer the patient, or is seeking to modify the activity to make performance of it possible, the content of the activity must first be analysed and evaluated. A preliminary analysis will consider the basic content of the activity in terms of, e.g.

- The kind(s) of performance needed to achieve the activity, e.g. cognitive, motor, interpersonal. (The headings for detailed analysis will depend on the approach being used.)
- Potential for engagement of patient interest and participation.
- Potential for therapeutic adaptation to meet treatment objectives.
- The degree of complexity of the activity.
- The positive or negative social or cultural associations.
- Whether the activity is structured or unstructured.
- Defining the tasks of which the activity is comprised.
- Analysing the sequence of task performance, and deciding whether this is fixed or flexible.

- Deciding whether the activity is familiar to the patient.
- Defining the tools, furniture, materials and environment required for completion of the activity.
- Defining and taking account of safety precautions or risk factors.
- Evaluation of whether or not to use the activity.

Activity synthesis. This invovles combining components of the activity and environment to produce a desired therapeutic outcome.

Adaptation of activity. The activity may be presented in unadapted form, or may be adapted to meet treatment goals. This is frequently tackled at the level of task adaptation (see later paragraph), since the adaptation required may differ from one stage of the activity to another. Typical adaptations are:

- *environmental*, e.g. location, setting, milieu, press.
- *equipment*, e.g. quantity of tools/materials, adaptation to tools.
- *social*, e.g. number of people, degree of interaction.
- *physical*, e.g. position, strength, range of movement.
- *cognitive*, e.g. complexity, sequence, need for instructions.
- *emotional*, e.g. interest, meaning, self-expression.
- *temporal*, e.g. duration, repetition.
- *structural*, e.g. order of tasks, omission of non-essential tasks.

Task analysis. This is breaking down the activity into tasks and the tasks into subtasks or processes, and analysing the general categories of motor, cognitive, perceptual or interactive skills required at each stage, or at any particular stage. This may include an analysis of specific movements and the types of muscle action or groups of muscles used to produce these. There are two main purposes for this exercise: either (1) to select an appropriate task to meet a therapeutic aim or objective, or (2) as a means of analysing the precise area of, or cause of a performance problem.

Selection of tasks for use as therapy may follow the sequence:

- Select task which offers potential to achieve the therapeutic objective. Consider motor, sensory, interactive, cognitive, symbolic, expressive factors.
- Analyse task, breaking it into component parts: subtasks, skills, subskills. Decide which portions of the task have therapeutic value and require emphasis/are irrelevant or inappropriate/are to be done by the patient/should be done for the patient.
- Decide need for adaptation of tools or materials; identify need for preparation.

Identification of the patient problem may follow the sequence:

- Observe patient performing task in realistic environment and context.
- Define and record problem area(s).
- Examine problem in subtask if required.
- Consider social/cultural factors if relevant.
- Consider roles of participant(s).
- Propose likely cause(s) of dysfunction, e.g. learning difficulty, developmental disorder, skill deficit, lack of practice, role rejection.

Grading — manipulating factors required in the performance of a task or activity to meet treatment goals. Grading typically includes changes to:

- sequence of task/components;
- size/shape of tools;
- position of tools/furniture/materials;
- quantity/specification of materials;
- speed/duration/repetition of performance;
- requirement for specific movements to perform task;
- strength required;
- perceptual components;
- cognitive components;
- simplicity/complexity;
- type of/quantity of instruction/demonstration/sample;
- the context (temporal, environmental, social, cultural) of the task;
- the location and content of the environment in which the task is performed;

Table 3 Examples of analytical structures of performance skills

Model of human occupation (Kielhofner)	Adaptation through occupation (Reed)	Adaptive skills (Mosey)
Interpersonal	Interpersonal	Sensory integration
Process	Intrapersonal	Cognitive function
Motor	Motor	Psychological function
Perceptual	Sensory	Social interaction
	Cognitive	

(It will be noted that the above lists are focused on performance skills and are not concerned with the analytical approach.)

- number of participants: requirement for interaction with others;
- degree of choice/creativity/decision taking/planning and problem solving.

Skill analysis. Conducting a full analysis of all the skills or subskills required to perform a particular task can be complex and time consuming. A task is performed as a gestalt, and 'unpacking' the components of performance or identifying the relationships between these and causes of dysfunction is not easy. The process is normally conducted by means of close observation combined with the use of knowledge of anatomy, physiology, perception, cognition, learning theory and theories of human interactions. It is usual to impose some kind of structure on such an analysis (see Table 3, above). Setting norms for performance is also difficult and is the object of research; unfortunately the 'super-fit' population frequently chosen for such studies renders the data inapplicable for most OT purposes.

Q There is extensive discussion in the literature of the criteria against which activities should be selected or rejected for use as therapy. Enduring arguments are:

1 Should OT only use purposeful, constructive activities? Are talking, thinking, imagining, relaxing, counselling, exercising, positioning, etc. legitimate OT tools?

2 How far should activities be adapted — is there a risk of 'adapting the activity out of existence'?

3 The therapist often values the process above the product — but the reverse may be true of the patient. Can both be satisfied?

4 How directive should the therapist be in the selection of therapeutic activities? How much choice should the patient have?

What is your opinion on the above questions? Make a few notes and then analyse what this indicates about your preferred model(s) and approach(es).

Is your answer influenced by the nature of the client group with which you are working? Discuss your answers with others. Do you believe there are 'right' and 'wrong' answers?

Summary of the core skills of occupational therapy

Managerial skills

Organizational
Financial
Recording
Research
Problem solving
Therapy/intervention planning★
Evaluation★

Interactive skills

Communication
Supervision
Teaching

Basic counselling
Basic group skills
Conscious use of self★

Therapeutic skills

Patient care
Observation
Application of knowledge★
Assessment★
Programme planning★
Application of technical and creative skills★
Application of therapeutic skills★
Analysis and adaptation of occupations★
Application of occupations as therapy★

★Primary core skills

SUGGESTED READING

As you might expect, references to the core skills of the profession can be found in almost every OT textbook.

Barnitt R 1990 Knowledge, skills and attitudes; what happened to thinking? British Journal of Occupational Therapy 53:11 450–456

Bumphrey E (ed) 1987 Occupational therapy in the community. Woodhead & Faulkner, Cambridge

Creek J (ed) 1990 Occupational therapy and mental health: principles, skills and practice. Churchill Livingstone, Edinburgh (section 5 Occupational therapy media and methods; section 7 Organization, administration & management)

Hopkins H L, Smith H D (eds) 1988 Willard & Spackman's occupational therapy, 7th edn. Lippincott, Philadelphia (ch 6 section 4 Activity; ch 8 section 4 Occupational behaviour; ch 17 ADL; ch 18 Work; ch 20 section 3 Leisure)

Kielhofner G (ed) 1985 A model of human occupation. Williams & Wilkins, Baltimore

Mosey A C 1981 Configuration of a profession. Raven Press, New York

Mosey A C 1986 Psychosocial components of occupational therapy. Raven Press, New York (ch 3 Performance components; ch 4 Occupational performance; ch 7 The non-human environment; ch 10 Purposeful activities; ch 11 Activity analysis and synthesis)

Pedretti L (ed) Occupational therapy: practice skills for physical dysfunction, 2nd edn. Mosby, New York

Sanderson S R, Reed K L 1980 Concepts of occupational therapy. Williams & Wilkins, Baltimore

Trombley C A 1983 Occupational therapy for physical dysfunction, 2nd edn. Williams & Wilkins, New York

Turner A (ed) 1991 The principles, skills & practice of occupational therapy. Churchill Livingstone, Edinburgh (ch 4 The OT process, part 2: Skills; ch 5 Management; ch 6 Activity analysis; ch 7 Assessment; ch 8 Life skills)

Young M, Quinn E 1991 Theories and practice of occupational therapy. Churchill Livingstone, Edinburgh (ch 7 Activity; ch 8 Work & leisure)

Bibliography

Abraham B 1988 The dilemmas of helping someone towards independence: an experiential account. British Journal of Occupational Therapy 51: 8 277–279

Allen C K 1985 Occupational therapy for psychiatric disorders: measurement and management of cognitive disabilities. Little Brown, Boston

Arnold M E, Penn B 1990 Expert systems and occupational therapy. British Journal of Occupational Therapy 53(9): 365–368

Ayres A J 1972 Sensory integration and learning disorders. Western Psychological Services, Los Angeles

Balint M 1984 The basic fault. Arrowsmith, Bristol

Bandura A 1977 Social learning theory. Prentice Hall, New Jersey

Barris R 1982 Environmental interactions, an extension of the model of human occupation. American Journal of Occupational Therapy 36(10):

Bigge M 1987 Learning theories for teachers, 4th edn. Harper & Row, New York

Bion W R 1961 Experience in groups. Tavistock Publications, London

Bobath B 1986 Adult hemiplegia: evaluation and treatment, 2nd edn. Heinemann, London

Bruce M A, Borg B 1987 Frames of reference in psychiatric occupational therapy. Slack, New Jersey

Bumphrey E (ed) 1987 Occupational therapy in the community. Woodhead & Faulkner, Cambridge

Burton J 1989 The model of human occupation and occupational therapy practice with elderly patients. Part 1: Characteristics of aging, Part 2: Application. British Journal of Occupational Therapy 52: 6 215–222

Cotton E, Kinsman R 1983 Conductive education for adult hemiplegia. Churchill Livingstone, Edinburgh

Creek J (ed) 1990 Occupational therapy and mental health: principles, skills and practice. Churchill Livingstone, Edinburgh

Douglas T 1976 Groupwork in practice. Tavistock Publications, London

Drouet V M 1986 Individual behavioural programme planning with long-stay schizophrenic patients. British Journal of Occupational Therapy 49(7): 227–232

Eagan G 1986 The skilled helper. Brooks Cole, California

Eggers O 1988 Occupational therapy in the rehabilitation of adult hemiplegia. Heinemann, London

Finlay L 1988 Occupational therapy practice in psychiatry. Croom Helm, London

Foulkes S H, Anthony E J 1965 Group psychotherapy: the analytical approach. Penguin, Harmondsworth

Gagné R M 1977 The conditions of learning and theory of instruction, 3rd edn. Holt Saunders, Eastbourne

Galley P M, Forster A L 1987 Human movement, 2nd edn. Churchill Livingstone, Edinburgh

Gerard B A, Boniface W J, Howe B H 1980

Interpersonal skills for health professionals. Reston, Virginia

Goodwill C J, Chamberlain M A (eds) 1988 Rehabilitation of the physically disabled adult. Croom Helm, London

Heap K 1979 Process and action in working with groups. Pergamon Press, Oxford

Hopkins H L, Smith H D (eds) 1988 Willard & Spackman's occupational therapy, 7th edn. Lippincott, Philadelphia

Howe M C, Schwartzberg S L 1986 A functional approach to group work in occupational therapy. Lippincott, Philadelphia

Hume C, Pullen M 1986 Rehabilitation in psychiatry. Churchill Livingstone, Edinburgh

Javetz, Katz 1989 Knowledgeability of theories of occupational therapy practitioners in Israel. American Journal of Occupational Therapy 43: 10

Jones M C 1983 Behaviour problems in handicapped children. Souvenir Press, London

Jones M 1960 An approach to occupational therapy. Butterworths, London

Jones M, Jay P (ed) 1977 An approach to occupational therapy, 3rd edn. Butterworths, London

Kielhofner G, Burke J P 1980 A model of human occupation, part 1. Conceptual framework and content. American Journal of Occupational therapy 34(9): 572–581

Kielhofner G 1980a A model of human occupation, part 2. Ontogenesis from the perspective of temporal adaptation. American Journal of Occupational Therapy 34(10): 657–663

Kielhofner G 1980b A model of human occupation, part 3. Benign and vicious cycles. American Journal of Occupational Therapy 34(11): 731–737

Kielhofner G, Burke J P, Igi C H 1980 A model of human occupation, part 4. Assessment and intervention. American Journal of Occupational Therapy 34(12): 777–778

Kielhofner G (ed) 1985 A model of human occupations. Williams & Wilkins, Baltimore

Kielhofner G 1988 The model of human occupation workbook. Workshops: London, Edinburgh, York

Kielhofner G, Nicol M 1989 The model of human occupation: a developing conceptual tool for clinicians. British Journal of Occupational Therapy 52: 6 210–214

Kirshenbaum H, Henderson V L (eds) 1990 Carl Rogers dialogues. Constable, London

Kirshenbaum H, Henderson V L (eds) 1990 The Carl Rogers reader. Constable, London

King L J 1974 A sensory integrative approach to schizophrenia. American Journal of Occupational Therapy 28: 529–536

Kings Fund Centre 1988 The problem orientated medical record (POMR): guidelines for therapists. Kings Fund Centre, London

Knowles M 1978 The adult learner: a neglected species, 3rd edn. Gulf, Houston

Llorens L A 1986 Activity analysis: agreement among factors in a sensory processing model. American Journal of Occupational Therapy 40:(2) 103–110

Lovell R B 1987 Adult learning. Croom Helm, London

Macdonald J 1990 The international course on conductive education at the Peto Andras State Institute for Conductive Education, Budapest. British Journal of Occupational Therapy 53:(7) 295–300

Maslow A H 1968 Towards a psychology of being. Van Nostrand, New York

Maslow A H 1970 Motivation and personality, Harper & Row, New York

McDonald E M 1964 Occupational therapy in rehabilitation, 2nd edn. Baillière Tindall, London

Mills D, Fraser C 1989 Therapeutic activities for the upper limb. Winslow Press, Bicester

Mocellin G 1988 A perspective on the principles and practice of occupational therapy. British Journal of Occupational Therapy 51: 14–7

Mosey A C 1968 Recapitulation of ontogenesis: a theory for the practice of occupational therapy. American Journal of Occupational Therapy 22:(5)

Mosey A C 1970 Three frames of reference for mental health. Slack, New Jersey

Mosey A C 1973 Activities therapy. Raven Press, New York

Mosey A C 1981 Occupational therapy: configuration of a profession. Raven Press, New York

Mosey A C 1986 Psychosocial components of occupational therapy. Raven Press, New York

Norkin C C, White J 1985 Measurement of joint motion. F A Davis, Philadelphia

Pedretti L (ed) 1985 Occupational therapy: practice skills for physical dysfunction, 2nd edn. C V Mosby, St Louis

Perry W G 1970 Forms of intellectual and ethical development in the college years: a scheme. Holt. Rinehart & Winston, New York

Priestly P et al 1978 Social skills and personal problem solving. Tavistock Publications, London

Reed K L 1984 Models of practice in occupational therapy. Williams & Wilkins, Baltimore

Remocker A J, Storch E T 1982 Action speaks louder. Churchill Livingstone, Edinburgh

Rimmer L 1982 Reality orientation principles and practice. Winslow Press, Bicester

Robertson E 1984 The role of the occupational therapist in a psychotherapeutic setting. British Journal of Occupational Therapy 47(4): 106–110

Rogers C 1983 Freedom to learn for the 80s. Charles E Merrill, Columbus, Ohio

Rogers C 1984 Client-centred therapy: its current practice, implications and theory. Houghton Miffin, Boston

Rogers C 1986 On becoming a person. Constable, London

Ross M, Burdick D 1981 Sensory integration. Slack, New Jersey

Sanderson S R, Reed K L 1980 Concepts of occupational therapy. Williams & Wilkins, Baltimore

Trombley C A 1983 Occupational therapy for physical dysfunction, 2nd edn. Williams & Wilkins, Baltimore

Turner A (ed) 1987 The practice of occupational therapy, 2nd edn. Churchill Livingstone, Edinburgh

Turner A (ed) 1991 The principles, skills and practice of occupational therapy. Churchill Livingstone, Edinburgh

Watts N 1990 Handbook of clinical teaching. Churchill Livingstone, Edinburgh

Watts F, Bennett D (eds) 1981 Principles of psychiatric rehabilitation. Wiley, Chichester

Weed L L 1968 Medical records that guide and teach. New England Journal of Medicine 278: 593–599

Weed L L 1969 Medical records, medical education and patient care. Western Reserve University, Cleveland

Wilcock A A 1986 Occupational therapy approaches to stroke. Churchill Livingstone, Edinburgh

Whittaker D S 1985 Using groups to help people. Routledge & Kegan Paul, London

Hogarth J 1978 Glossary of health care terminology. World Health Organization, Copenhagen

Willson M 1984 Occupational therapy in short term psychiatry, 2nd edn. Churchill Livingstone, Edinburgh

Willson M 1987 Occupational therapy in long term psychiatry, 2nd edn. Churchill Livingstone, Edinburgh

Wing J K, Morris B (eds) 1981 Handbook of psychiatric rehabilitation. Oxford University Press, Oxford

Yallom I D 1975 Theory and practice of group psychotherapy. Basic Books, New York

Yallom I D 1983 In-patient group psychotherapy. Basic Books, New York

Young M 1984 Models of practice for occupational therapy. British Journal of Occupational Therapy 47(12): 381–382

Young M, Quinn E 1991 Theories and practice of occupational therapy. Churchill Livingstone, Edinburgh

Yule W, Carr J Behaviour modification for the mentally handicapped. Croom Helm, London

Zoltan B, Seiv E, Freishtat B 1986 Perceptual and cognitive dysfunction in the adult stroke patient, 2nd edn. Slack, New Jersey

Glossary

Note

The Glossary includes words defined in the text, and words used in connection with models and professional practice. It does not include medical or psychological terms which may be found readily in specialist dictionaries, but a few terms which may be difficult to find, or are notoriously confusing, are defined. Where there are two meanings, or where several, differing definitions exist, the alternatives are given.

Sources of definitions

Proliferating lists of definitions are of no use to the student, or to the profession. Where clear definitions exist which are compatible with the text, I have a used these, and sources are indicated as shown in the code below. Those marked (RH) are my own.

(Cr)   Creek J (ed) 1990 Occupational therapy and mental health: principles, skills and practice. Churchill Livingstone, Edinburgh

(WS)   Hopkins H L, Smith H D (eds) 1988 Willard and Spackman's occupational therapy, 7th edn. Lippincott, Philadelphia

(Kh)   Kielhofner G 1988 The model of human occupation workbook. Workshops: London, Edinburgh, York

(Lov)   Lovell R B 1987 Adult learning. Croom Helm, London

(SR)   Sanderson S R, Reed K L 1980 Concepts of occupational therapy. Williams and Wilkins, Baltimore

(COD)   Skyes J B (ed) 1982 The concise Oxford dictionary, 7th edn. Clarendon Press, Oxford

(WHO)   Hogarth J 1978 Glossary of health care terminology. World Health Organization, Copenhagen

( )   *Other authors given in brackets.*

GENERAL GLOSSARY

Algorithm   A diagrammatic method of illustrating the stages and alternative decisions at each stage in a process.   (RH)

Autonomy   Personal freedom; freedom of the will. (COD)
The ability to act or perform according to one's own volition or direction.   (SR)
Quality of being self governing and self determining.   (WS)

Behaviour   Any action or actions of the individual.   (Lov)
(Molar behaviour: the action of the whole organism.)

Behaviourism   Study of human actions by analysis into stimulus and response.   (COD)
A branch of psychology which attempts to discover the laws that describe behaviour by relying exclusively on observable data.   (Lov)

Cognitive   Relating to the conscious mental processes required for knowing and understanding, such as perception, memory, imagination, judgement, reasoning and problem solving.   (RH)

Concept   A system of learned responses which enables us to organize and interpret data.   (Lov)
Idea of a class of objects.   (COD)
A general idea or meaning usually mediated by a work, symbol or sign.   (SR)

Competency   The ability to perform skills to the level of efficiency required by physical, psychological and social health.   (SR)

Countertransference   Conscious or unconscious responses of the therapist to the patient, determined by the therapist's need; transferred feelings, not necessarily relevant to the real situation.   (WS)

Defence mechanism   Unconscious intrapsychic process, e.g. denial, introjection, projection, rationalization.   (WS)

Determinism   Doctrine that human action is not free, but determined by motives regarded as external forces acting on the will.   (COD)

Development   The progressive and continuous change in shape, function and integration of the body from birth to death.   (SR)

Disability   Loss or impairment of one or more bodily organs, with corresponding functional loss.   (COD)
The reduction of functional ability to lead a fruitful daily life. It is the result not only of mental and/or physical impairment, but also of the individual's adjustment to this.   (WHO)
Note: This term must be considered along with impairment, handicap and incapacity. The various terms have not always been clearly distinguished from one another. In general English usage, disability and handicap are often used interchangeably, and there is a tendency to equate both terms with the more severe and obvious conditions. A logical sequence might be:

Impairment   The basic pathological condition. An impairment may be so minor as not to interfere materially with functional ability, or it may be possible to correct or restore function. If an impairment is major, and not capable of correction, it will produce:

Disability   The loss or reduction of functional ability. The effect of this will depend on the individual's personal circumstances and requirements. It may well amount to:

Handicap   The disadvantage or restriction of activity caused by disability.

(WHO)

Divergent thinking   A cognitive operation in which the subject thinks in different directions. The quality of divergent thought is judged in terms of the quantity, variety and originality of the ideas produced.   (Lov)

Dualism   Theory recognizing two independent principles — mind and matter.   (COD)

Dyadic interaction   *Of skills:* Abilities in relationships to peers, subordinates and authority figures; demonstrating trust, respect and warmth; perceiving and responding to needs and feelings of others; engaging in and sustaining interdependent relationships; communicating feelings.   (SR)

Eclectic   Borrowing   freely   from   various sources.   (COD)

Ecology (human)   Study of interaction of persons with their environment.   (COD)

Empirical   Founded on practical experience but not proved scientifically; based on observable fact or objective experience.   (WS)

Environment   Composit of all external forces and influences affecting the development and maintenance of an individual.   (WS)

Ethnographic   Research techniques developed for social or anthropological studies.   (RH)

Evaluation 1. *Of therapy*: Systematic appraisal of effectiveness. (RH)
2. The process of collecting and interpreting data obtained through observation, interview, record review or testing. (SR)

Existentialism Philosophical theory emphasizing existence of the individual person as a free and responsible agent, determining his own development. (COD)

Experiential learning A view that all learning is best gained by direct experience, which must be meaningful to the learner. (RH)

Feedback Modification or control of a process or system by its results and effects, especially by difference between desired and actual result. (COD)
Information about the consequences of the actions taken by a person performing a skill. (Lov)
The process of returning to a system information concerning output and its consequences. (Kh)

Gestalt Perceived organized whole that is more than the sum of its parts. (COD)

Habilitation The encouragement and stimulation of the development and acquisition of skills and functions not previously attained. (SR)

Handicap Having less than normal ability or having an anatomical or functional defect which makes it difficult for one to compete with one's peers. (SR) (See also, Disability.)

Heuristic Quality that encourages further discovery or investigation. (WS)

Hierarchy The arrangement of parts of a system into interconnected lower and higher components, in which higher components can command lower ones and lower ones can constrain the higher. (Kh)

Holistic *Of therapy:* A conscious attempt to view all aspects of a client's problem or situation as a gestalt, and to treat all aspects accordingly. (RH)

Humanism System which views man as a responsible and progressive intellectual being. (COD)
A system of beliefs and a theoretical approach that is concerned with what it means to become fully human. (Cr)

Hypothesis Proposition made as a basis for reasoning without assumption of its truth; supposition made as a starting point for further investigation from known facts. (COD)

Illuminative study One which recounts subjective personal experience with a view to providing insights into causes, processes and the effectiveness of procedures. (RH)

Information processing *In cognitive psychology:* The mental processes required to store, retrieve and make use of information. (RH)

Input Information entering a system from the environment. (RH)

Kinesiology The study of human movement. (RH)

Mechanistic *Relates to:* Doctrine that all natural phenomena, including life, allow mechanical explanation by physics and chemistry. (COD)
The tendency to see all phenomena as machine-like in their operations. (Kh)

Modelling Setting an example (usually, of social behaviour) for imitation. (RH)

Monism Any of the theories which deny the duality of matter and mind. (COD)

Naturalistic method Techniques of research conducted in normal environments without artificial controls. (RH)

Object relations The ability of the person to invest feelings and emotions in other persons or objects. (SR)

Ontogenesis Origin and development of an individual. (COD)
Development of an individual over the passage of time. (RH)

Organismic A view of reality which emphasizes the subjective, interactive and holistic nature of human experience. (RH)

Output The product of the processes of a system. (RH)
Action of the system which produces a change in the environment; mental, physical and social aspects of occupation. (Kh)

Perception Mental process by which intellectual, sensory and emotional data are organized meaningfully; the process of conscious recognition and interpretation of sensory stimuli. (WS)

Phenomenological Relating to the study of *phenomena* — things which are perceived and reported as part of conscious subjective experience. (RH)

Philosophy Seeking after wisdom or knowledge, especially that which deals with ultimate reality or the most general causes and principles of things and ideas, and human perception and knowledge of them. (COD)
A critique and analysis of fundamental beliefs as they come to be conceptualized and formalized. (SR)

Physiology Science of functions and phenomena of living organisms and their parts. (COD)

Problem oriented medical records (POMR) A system for recording problems affecting a patient and planning and organizing action to resolve these. (RH)

Problem solving Refers to skill and performance in identifying and organizing solutions to difficulties. (SR)

Profession An occupation characterized by a defined body of knowledge and expertise, whose practitioners espouse a code of ethics and responsible conduct in relation to their clients. (RH)

Proprioception Appreciation of position, balance and changes in equilibrium of a body part during movement as a result of stimulus to receptors within body tissue such as muscle, tendons and joints. (WS)

Psychoanalysis A therapeutic system for the treatment of mental disorder based on the principles of analytical psychology, aimed at investigating interaction of conscious and un-

conscious elements in the mind, and bringing the latter into consciousness. (RH)

Psychotherapy Treatment of mental disorder in which a trained person interacts with the patient on the basis of a therapeutic contract; treatment is based on communication. (WS)

Psychology Science of the nature, functions and phenomena of the human mind. (COD)

Rehabilitation The restoration of a person's skills and functions to the fullest physical, mental, social, vocational and economic usefulness of which that person is capable. (SR)
Restoration to a disabled individual of maximum independence, commensurate with his limitations by developing his residual capacities. (WS)
The combined and coordinated use of medical, social, educational and vocational measures for training or retraining the individual to the highest possible level of functional ability. (WHO)

Rehabilitative services Those activities and procedures designed to assist a physically or mentally disabled individual to achieve or maintain the highest attainable level of function through an evaluation and treatment programme providing, under physician direction, one or a combination of medical, paramedical, psychological, social and vocational services determined by the needs of the patient. (WHO)

Self-actualization The capacity of the individual to achieve a life which fulfils potentials and offers satisfaction and personal meaning. (RH)

SOAP Heading used in problem oriented medical records: Subjective; Objective; Analysis; Plan. (RH)

Standardized *Of assessments:* One which provides for measurement against a criterion or norm. The assessment must be performed according to the testing protocol. (SR)

Systems theory The basis for the study of the operation of systems. Systems may be described as 'hard', i.e. of a fixed, mechanical nature; or 'soft', i.e. changing, dynamic interactions between people and environments. The operation of a system is usually described in terms of input, output, throughput and feedback. (RH)

Taxonomy Principles of classification. (COD) (Especially used in botany, biology and education.)

Teleological Purposeful; relating to the view that developments are due to the purpose or design that is served by them. (COD)

Temporal Of, in, or denoting time. (COD)

Theory A system of assumptions, accepted principles and rules of procedure devised to analyse, predict or otherwise explain the nature or behaviour of a specific set of phenomena. (SR) Set of logically interrelated statements used to explain observed events. A proposed explanation whose status is still conjectural, in contrast to well established propositions that are regarded as reporting matters of fact. (WS)

Throughput Material which is put through a system and processed by it. The transformation of imported information and energy to another form and its incorporation into the structure of the system, resulting in structural maintenance and change. (Kh)

Topological Relating to the study of geometrical properties and spatial relations unaffected by continuous change of shape or size of figures. (COD) (The shape is capable of mutation without losing the essential relationships of its features.)

Transference *In psychoanalysis*: Projection of feelings, thoughts or wishes on to another who has come to represent someone from the past; inappropriate feelings applied in present context. (WS)

Validated *Of assessment*: A standardized test whose results are statistically reliable within given parameters, as proved by controlled research. (RH)

TERMS USED IN OCCUPATIONAL THERAPY

Activity Purposeful behaviour designed to achieve a desired goal. A specific action, function or sphere of action that involves learning or doing by direct experience. (SR)

Activity programme A programme designed to encourage individual and/or group participation through organized events for the purpose of maintaining or improving skills, roles or interactions. (RH)

Adaptation 1. Any change in structure, form or habits of an organism to suit a new environment. Those changes experienced by an individual which lead to adjustment. (WS)
2. An alteration made by a therapist to an environment or an object in order to provide therapy or to improve the client's ability to function. (RH)

Adaptive behaviour The integration of skill areas with socially accepted values to accomplish occupations and tasks. (SR)

Aim A brief statement of the general purpose which treatment or intervention will be planned to achieve. (RH)

Approach A mental set derived from a synthesis of related techniques and methods which leads the therapist to select particular assessments, treatment techniques or a style of relationship appropriate to the needs of the patient/client. (RH)

Assessment The process of collecting information, including subjective and objective data which are relevant to the preparation of an intervention plan. (RH)

Core skills Basic components of professional practice, managerial, interactive and therapeutic which remain relatively constant although adapted by the use of frames of reference, models and approaches. (RH)

Diversional activities Those designed to alleviate boredom and to provide an enjoyable interest, without specific therapeutic intent. (RH)

Dysfunction A temporary or chronic inability to engage in the roles, relationships and occupations expected of a person of a comparable age, sex and culture. (RH)
Inability to maintain the self within the environment at a satisfactory standard because of lack of skills necessary for coping with the current situation. (Cr)

Environmental press The effect of environmental factors such as objects, tasks, people and culture, in promoting or suppressing engagement in particular activities or interactions. (RH)

Facilitation 1. *Of groups:* Helpful, nondirective leadership style. (RH)
2. *Of neurodevelopmental techniques:* Specific treatment which promotes sensory motor integration and the recovery or development of normal patterns of movement. (RH)

Frame of reference Belief system based on conceptual models; in therapy, organized basis of theory, delineation of function and dysfunction, evaluation and treatment approaches, postulates regarding change. (WS)
A set of interrelated, internally consistent concepts, definitions and postulates derived from or compatible with empirical data, providing a systematic description or proscription for particular designs of the environment for the purpose of facilitating evaluation and effecting change. (Mosey)
A set of basic assumptions necessary to determine the subject matter to be studied and the orientation towards such study. (SR)
The principles behind practice; the organization of knowledge in a particular field to permit description of the relationships between facts and concepts. (Cr)
A statement of facts, theories and hypotheses in a particular field of study, which provides a coherent basis for therapy. (RH)

Functional ability The skill to perform activities in a normal or accepted manner. (SR)

Grading Measurable increasing or decreasing of activity, graded by length of time, size, degree of strength required or amount of energy expended. (SR)

Habituation subsystem A collection of images which trigger and divide the performance of routine patterns of behaviour. Two sets of these images exist and interrelate in guiding everyday behaviour; they are referred to as habits and roles. (Kh)

Interpersonal *Of skills:* Those which are used for interactions between people. The level, quality and/or degree of dyadic and group interaction skills. (WS)

Intervention Action by the therapist on behalf of the client/patient. The process of putting the plan into action and carrying it out. (WS)

Intrapersonal *Of skills:* Those which operate within the mind and emotions of the individual. (RH)
The level, quality and/or degree of self-identity, self-concept and coping skills. (WS)

Meaningfulness *Of activities:* The individual's predisposition to find importance, security, sense of worth and purpose in certain forms of occupations. (Kh)

Medium An agency or activity through which something is accomplished. An intervening substance through which something is transmitted or carried on. In OT, an activity or task having therapeutic potential. (SR)

Modality A therapeutic agent/activity; the application of a therapeutic agent. (SR) (syn. Medium)

Model A set of ideas derived from various fields of study which are organized to form a synthesis and integration of elements of theory and practice. (RH)
A representational tool which orders, categorizes and simplifies complex phenomena; describes the organization among parts. (Kh)
A simplified representation of the structure and content of a phenomenon or system that describes or explains the complex relationships between concepts within the system. (Cr)

Occupation A cluster of activities described by a specific title and defined general purpose, related to work, leisure, self care or social role. (RH)
Activity or task which engages a person's resources of time and energy. Specifically: self-maintenance, productivity and leisure. (SR)
The human being's interaction with the environment which arises out of an innate urge towards exploration and mastery and the consequent ability to symbolize; the essence of human existence and adaptation. (Kh)
Any goal directed activity that has meaning for the individual and is composed of skills and values. (Cr)

Occupational behaviour Organization and action based on skills, knowledge and attitude to make functioning possible in life roles. (Reilly)

Occupational therapy The treatment of physical and psychiatric conditions through specific selected activities in order to help people to reach their maximum level of function in all aspects of daily life. (WFOT)
The restoration or maintenance of optimal functional independence and life satisfaction through the analysis and use of selected occupations that enable the individual to develop the adaptive skills required to support his life roles. (Cr)
The prescription of occupations, interactions and environmental adaptations to enable the individual to regain, develop or retain the occupational skills and roles required to maintain personal well being and to achieve meaningful personal goals and relationships appropriate to the relevant social and cultural setting. (RH)

Objective A precise statement of the purpose and outcome of therapy. (RH)

Paradigm Accepted examples of scientific practice which include law, theory appreciation and instrumentation and which represent a radically new conceptualization of the phenomena. (Kuhn)
A consensus of the most fundamental beliefs or assumptions of a field. The occupational therapy paradigm is the field's means of defining human beings and their problems in a way which suggests and provides a rationale for courses of action to solve them. (Kh)
An agreed body of theory, explaining and rationalizing professional unity and practice, that incorporates all the profession's concerns, concepts and expertise and guides values and commitments. (Cr)

Performance skills Skills required for successful performance of the roles that are assumed by individuals in their lives. (WS)

Performance subsystem Collection of images and biological components which are used in the production of skilled behaviour. (Kh)

Personal causation Self-perception of effectiveness within the environment. (Kh)
The individual's capacity to intitiate action with the intent to affect the environment. (Cr)

Role A social or occupational identity which directs the individual's social, cultural and occupational behaviour and relationships. Individuals typically require the capacity to carry out a variety of roles at any point in life. (RH)

Skill A specific ability, or integrated set of abilities, (e.g. motor, sensory, cognitive or perceptual) learnt and practised to a standard required for the effective performance of a task or subtask. (RH)

Subskill A primary component of a skill. (RH)

Subtask A non-reducible component of a task. (RH)

Task A stage in or component of an activity. (RH)

Techniques The body of specialized procedures and methods used in treatment. (RH)

Volition subsystem An interrelated set of energizing and symbolic components which together determine conscious choices. The energizing component is a generalized urge for exploration and mastery. The symbolic components are images (beliefs, recollections, convictions, expectations) which include values, personal causation and interests. (Kh)

OCCUPATIONAL THERAPY TECHNIQUES

Note

The definitions given below are my own, unless otherwise stated. This is not intended as a comprehensive list, but as an indication of some commonly used techniques and an explanation of some of the terms used in the text which may be unfamiliar to you.

Some of the techniques are primary core skills which all therapists should possess and use. These are marked (CS). Others are those of which a newly qualified therapist may be expected to have a basic knowledge: these have been indicated (B). Those marked (S) are more specialist techniques. A newly qualified therapist may have an understanding of the basic principles, but the technique would would normally require additional experience and training and would be used by a senior practitioner, or under close supervision.

Activity analysis (CS)   Dissection of an activity into its component tasks and the evaluation of therapeutic potential and relevance to the treatment plan.

Activity synthesis (CS)   Combining and adapting components of an activity with components of the environment to assess performance, enhance skills or produce a desired therapeutic outcome.

Adaptation to activity (CS)   Modification of features such as sequence, complexity, positioning, location, use of tools, construction of equipment, etc. to meet treatment objectives or to improve performance. ·

Anxiety management (S)   Techniques having a cognitive and/or behavioural basis, used to help clients to monitor and control personal anxiety levels.

Assertion training (S)   Techniques which enable the individual to appreciate personal individuality and worth, to recognize personal feelings and needs and to express these in a socially acceptable manner. Training often employs group techniques and role play.

Behaviour modification (S)   The use of structured programmes, including reinforcement, to modify behaviour, either by removing an unproductive, injurious or antisocial behaviour, or by promoting positive behaviours.

Behavioural rehearsal (S)   A cognitive technique in which the client acts out and practises behaviours which are found to be difficult or stressful before attempting them in reality.

Biofeedback (S)   Technique in which the patient is made aware of unconscious or involuntary physiological processes, and learns to control them.   (WS)

Chaining (B)   Technique of teaching behaviour patterns by giving reinforcement for individual components of a behaviour, which may be learnt separately and then linked to form a whole. *Backward chaining* is a form of errorless learning in which a task or behaviour is taught by commencing at the point of completion and working backwards to the start.

Counselling (S)   The use of client centred techniques to enable the client to identify problems, feelings or conflicts and to reach solutions or decisions.

Desensitization (S)   Use of progressive exposure of the patient in a safe environment to a stimulus which provokes acute anxiety or other negative reaction until the point is reached where the patient can tolerate the stimulus without becoming dysfunctional.

Environmental analysis (CS)   Observation of features in the physical or social environment and interpretation of their significance, for patient performance, or therapy.

Environmental adaptation (CS)   Changing the physical or social features of an environment to enhance performance, promote or restrict a behaviour, or provide therapy.

Energy conservation (S)   Techniques including time management, time and motion study, problem solving and environmental planning, enabling a patient to make maximum functional use of limited potential for energy expenditure.

Errorless learning (S) Techniques (cognitive/behavioural) which teach concepts or skills by presenting material or instruction in such a way that the possibility of failure by the learner is eliminated.

Gaming (S) The use of scenarios, tasks, or problem solving exercises to provide groups of people with personal experience of group processes, decision making mechanisms, leadership styles, or the effects of emotions, attitudes and preconceptions.

Guided fantasy (S) Techniques in which a group leader, by means of words, images or music, provides stimulus for each individual to construct mental images, stories or journeys leading to insightful exploration of personal symbols, fantasies, desire, emotions or choices.

Home adaptations (B) The design and provision of physical alterations to an individual's home in order to promote independent living.

Homework (S) A term used in some cognitive techniques where a patient is given tasks to do at home, usually involving a record of results and personal reactions during and after the process.

Interviews (B) Techniques include formal, informal, structured and unstructured methods; interviews may be used to obtain information or to negotiate aims and objectives or to evaluate courses of action.

Industrial therapy (S) Use of industrial work processes — frequently packing, assembly work or clerical work — in a simulation of a realistic work environment, with nominal pay, to assess, promote or retrain work skills.

Joint protection (S) Instructing patients in ways of managing personal, domestic or work activities in a manner which reduces or eliminates potentially damaging stresses on vulnerable joints. Particularly used in the management of arthritic conditions.

Milieu therapy (S) A psychotherapeutic term meaning the modification of a physical and social environment, such as that provided by a therapeutic community, for treatment purposes.

Mobility training (B) Instruction of a patient in the use of mobility equipment and wheelchairs.

Neurodevelopmental techniques (B/S) Techniques used in the treatment of sensori-motor disorders which are based on the use of techniques such as reflex inhibition, positioning, and sensory stimulation (e.g. Bobath; Rood; PNF).

Orthotics (B/S) Assessment for, design of, and production and fitting of orthoses (splints) for functional or supportive purposes, often for the upper limb.

Perceptual training (B) Techniques designed to train or re-educate perceptual functions such as discriminations of size, form, colour, laterality, by repeated practice.

Portage (S) A developmentally based programme constructed by a therapist enabling a parent of a handicapped child to work with the child at home, using play and care activities to achieve defined goals.

Prosthetic training (B/S) Techniques of instructing patients in the use of upper and lower limb prostheses following amputation.

Projective techniques (B/S) The use of creative media, especially art, music, modelling and writing in a manner which encourages the patient to explore personal experiences, symbols and feelings.

Psychodrama (S) The use of dramatic techniques, e.g. role play, improvization, mime, to construct or reconstruct scenarios of significance to the participants, or to engage them in experiences which will enable them to explore life themes, emotions, thoughts, reactions, relationships or defensive and coping mechanisms.

Reality orientation (B) Used with dementing or brain damaged individuals to cue them into awareness of current time, place, persons and circumstances. Can involve '24 hour' and 'classroom' techniques.

Relaxation (B) Various methods involving techniques of voluntary physical control designed to produce physical and mental relaxation and relieve the effects of stress or anxiety.

Reminiscence therapy (nostalgia therapy) (B) Techniques used with dementing individuals or very elderly people in which objects from the past — photos, music, clothes, tools, etc. — are used as triggers for discussion and reflection and the sharing of personal experiences and memories, enhancing individuality.

Room management techniques (S) A means of providing individual attention to members of a large group for short periods, making best use of available staff and their skills, and the possibly limited attention span of participants. Typically, one person acts as 'room manager', coordinating therapy, whilst another looks after physical care needs, or disturbances, and one or more others spend a few minutes with each group member in turn, working for a predetermined objective.

Role play (B/S) Use of dramatic techniques and improvization to enable patients to act out roles or situations which they wish to explore, either to gain insight into difficulties, or to improve coping skills.

Sensory re-education (B/S) Usually carried out to restore sensitivity and discrimination of touch in the hand following peripheral nerve injury; the patient is trained to recognize a variety of progressively finer and more similar textures by touch alone.

Skill analysis (CS) Analysis of a skill to identify the subskills required for its performance.

Social modelling (B) Shaping behaviour or attitudes by enabling the learner to observe others performing competently and gaining suitable rewards or approval for such performance.

Social skills training (B) Educational programmes designed to improve skills of interaction and acceptable social behaviour. May use social modelling, role play and behavioural rehearsal.

Stress management (B/S) A variety of cognitive and behavioural techniques used to enable the individual to recognize signs of personal stress and to adopt positive preventative and coping strategies to reduce this.

Task analysis (CS) Breaking a task down into a sequence of subtasks and identifying the skills, or physical movements or interactions required at each stage.

Token economy (S) A form of behavioural modification in which the patient is rewarded for fulfilling a specified behavioural contract by 'tokens', which are usually tradeable for goods or privileges.

Appendix 1

The following table indicates some of the general areas of assessment, and the types of techniques used within each of the models and approaches described in this book.

Table of assessment techniques used in models and approaches

MODEL/APPROACH	ASSESSMENT General areas (e.g.'s)	Techniques
PHYSIOLOGICAL		
Neurodevelopmental approach	Motor patterns — spasticity; flaccidity Coordination Sensory deficits Apraxia Reflexes Proprioception Perceptual deficits Integration of sensory/motor function Chronological developmental stages	Observation and physical examination; check-lists and record charts; unstructured interview
Biomechanical approach	Range of movement Strength of movement Speed of movement Dexterity/coordination Stamina Sensation Hand function — prehension Functional limitation Need for orthosis Use of prosthesis Need for adaptive equipment	Observation and physical examination; use of physical measurement equipment; check-lists and record charts; unstructured or structured interview
BEHAVIOURAL	Performance skills, e.g. personal care skills; communication skills; social skills; physical skills Abnormal responses, e.g. challenging behaviour; self mutilation; aggression	A variety of standardized validated tests of performance and behaviour. Several such tests are marketed, but some are only available for use by OTs with special training. Informal tests with a behavioural format may be used; structured interview

continued overleaf

MODEL/APPROACH	ASSESSMENT General areas (e.g.'s)	Techniques
COGNITIVE	IQ Perception of objects, time, place, person Memory Attention/concentration Problem solving Organization Attitudes and Values Flexibility/rigidity Agnosia Intellectual abilities—numeracy; literacy Personality traits	There are many validated tests but therapists may need special training to use some. Tests are usually structured — check-lists; record charts. Several OT tests are available (e.g. Rivermead, COTNAB). Full cognitive assessment is best performed by a clinical psychologist; structured interview
PSYCHODYNAMIC		
Analytical approach	Perception of self Perception of others Object relations Use of symbols	Standardized assessments are not generally used by occupational therapists in this approach. Some tests use projective, associative and symbolic media. Personality tests can only be used by therapists with special training; unstructured interview
Interactive approach	Perception of self Perception of others Communication skills Assertion skills Level of stress Level of anxiety Social skills Reactions and interactions in groups	Some standardized tests are available for skills assessment; otherwise observation of the patient in interactive settings is used; unstructured interview
HUMANIST	Assessment by a person external to the client is largely irrelevant within this model, but self assessment tests may be used to help the client to define problem areas or to formulate future goals. Interviews use client centred, reflective techniques.	
REHABILITATION	Rehabilitative assessments are functionally based and aimed at identifying deficits and charting recovery. Assessments tend to be related to either the chosen approach or technique, or to a specific occupational area — see elsewhere in this table. Structured or unstructured interviews.	
DEVELOPMENTAL	Chronological versus actual developmental levels in performance skills — motor, sensory, perceptual, cognitive, interactive	Tests are frequently standardized and many formal tests are sold for use in paediatrics; structured or unstructured interviews
EDUCATIONAL	Assessment of educational attainment, except at a very basic level, is not within the remit of an occupational therapist and the client should be referred to an educationalist or educational psychologist. Tests used by occupational therapists in this context tend to be cognitive, behavioural or occupational (see elsewhere in this table).	
PROBLEM SOLVING	It is not possible to specify assessment areas within this model because they will be chosen to relate to the nature of the patient's problem. Any of those listed might be appropriate — other than those highly specific ones which imply that one has already chosen to work within another model.	

MODEL/APPROACH	ASSESSMENT General areas (e.g.'s)	Techniques
ADAPTIVE SKILLS	Assessment of developmental level in six performance areas: Sensory integration Cognition Perception Dyadic interaction Group interaction Self identity	Standardized tests devised for use within the model; interviews
ADAPTATION THROUGH OCCUPATIONS	Evaluation of physical, psychosocial, developmental and environmental problems. Skill development Chained behaviour Information skills Problem solving skills	Standardized tests devised for use within the model; interviews
HUMAN OCCUPATIONS	Evaluation of dysfunction within the volition, habituation and performance subsystems. Evaluation of environment. Evaluation of performance in the occupational areas of work, leisure and self care. Specific assessments Values/attitudes Interests Perceptions of control Use of/perceptions of time Habits and organization Roles Performance skills: interpersonal; process; motor; perceptual	Standardized tests devised for use within the model — some are self-rating; structured interviews
OCCUPATIONAL AREAS	Some OT assessments are related to occupational areas rather than to a model, although probably used within the context of one.	
Activities of daily living	Performance skills in ADL, e.g. personal care — toilet, washing, dressing; eating Domestic activities — cooking, cleaning, shopping Mobility Communication Need for adaptive equipment Home assessment	Observation; check-lists; record forms; performance tests; some standardized tests; interviews
Work	Skills, knowledge, attitudes and habits required for work. Specific, e.g. Work tolerance Time keeping Work related skills — motor; cognitive; sensory; interpersonal Numeracy; literacy Assessment of work place environment Work aptitudes	Observation; performance tests; Check-lists and rating scales. Some standardized tests; structured and unstructured interviews. Full work aptitude assessment is best referred to an occupational psychologist or for vocational guidance.

continued overleaf

MODEL/APPROACH	ASSESSMENT General areas (e.g.'s)	Techniques
Leisure	Skills, interests and attitudes related to leisure. Attitudes/values Use of time/ability to plan Interests inventory Self perception Mapping of leisure participation	Questionnaires and check-lists, often self-rating; structured and unstructured interviews

Useful exercises in connection with this section:

1 List the assessment procedures which you are currently using. Does the list indicate a preferred model?
2 Do you use/have you seen in use any standardized or validated tests?
3 Obtain a selection of OT assessment forms and procedures and take a critical look at these. How clear are they? Do they look professionally presented? How valid do you think the results of the assessment can be considered to be?
4 If you think that a form or procedure could be improved, how would you do this? Try making up a new version.

Appendix 2

EXAMPLES OF COMMONLY USED OCCUPATIONAL THERAPY MEDIA (ADULTS)

Expressive and projective media

- art
- collage
- clay work
  (modelling, pottery)
- creative writing
- drama
- dance
- literature
- masks
- mime

- music
- poetry
- puppetry

Leisure activities

- ball games
- cognitive games
- computer games
- flower arranging
- keep fit exercises
- music
- outings
- parties
- puzzles
- quizzes
- remedial games
- riding
- singing
- social activities
- swimming
- team games
- video games

Technical activities

- assembly work
- computer operating
- carpentry
- clerical work
- horticulture
- metalwork
- photography
- printing
- screenprinting
- video

Constructive activities and crafts

- batik
- beadwork
- canework
- candlemaking
- carving
- crochet
- dressmaking
- embroidery
- enamelling
- fabric printing
- fretwork
- jewellery
- knitting
- macrame
- marbling
- origami
- pyrography
- rugmaking
- sewing
- stencils
- stool seating
- tapestry
- weaving

Domestic and self care activities

- bathing
- beauty care

- child care
- cooking
- DIY
- dressing
- dressmaking
- driving
- eating
- gardening
- hair care and
  grooming
- pet care
- personal toilet
- laundering
- housework
- shopping
- travelling
- walking

Index